COMPLEX REGIONAL PAIN SYNDROME

(CRPS) AND AMPUTATION:

A DIFFICULT DECISION TO MAKE

Volume IV

Alaa Abd-Elsayed M.D., MPH, FASA and Eric M. Phillips

First edition, 2021 – Volume IV

ISBN: 9798717555821

Other books published by authors:

Alaa Abd-Elsayed

- Chronic Pain: The Patient and Family Journey
- If the Savior is not Safe, How Can He Save?
- Pain: A Review Guide
- Infusion Therapy for Pain, Headache and Related Conditions
- Complex Regional Pain Syndrome (CRPS): Patients' Perspective of Living in Chronic Pain: Volume 1
- Complex Regional Pain Syndrome (CRPS): Patients' Perspective of Living in Chronic Pain: Volume 1-Picture eBook
- Complex Regional Pain Syndrome (CRPS): Patients' Perspective of Living in Chronic Pain: Volume II
- Complex Regional Pain Syndrome (CRPS): Patients' Picture eBook Guide: Volume II
- What is CRPS? A Helpful Guide to Teach Children About Complex Regional Pain Syndrome (CRPS): Volume III
- Complex Regional Pain Syndrome (CRPS): Patients' Picture eBook Guide: Volume III

Eric M. Phillips

- Complex Regional Pain Syndrome (CRPS): Patients' Perspective of Living in Chronic Pain: Volume 1
- Complex Regional Pain Syndrome (CRPS): Patients' Perspective of Living in Chronic Pain: Volume 1-Picture eBook
- Don't Diet: Change Your Eating Habits - Proper Eating for Good Health
- Complex Regional Pain Syndrome (CRPS): Patients' Perspective of Living in Chronic Pain: Volume II
- Complex Regional Pain Syndrome (CRPS): Patients' Picture eBook Guide: Volume II
- What is CRPS? A Helpful Guide to Teach Children About Complex Regional Pain Syndrome (CRPS): Volume III
- Complex Regional Pain Syndrome (CRPS): Patients' Picture eBook Guide: Volume III

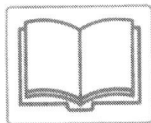

The MG Academy LLC

Dedication

To my parents, my wife and my two beautiful kids Maro and George.

To all CRPS patients.

Alaa Abd-Elsayed

Dedication

To my loving parents, Janet and my late father Leonard (Lenny) for all their love, and support.

To my beautiful and supportive wife Mercedes, her three children and her grandson.

To my mentor, teacher and greatest friend the late Doctor Hooshang Hooshmand.

To all CRPS patients worldwide.

Eric M. Phillips

TABLE OF CONTENTS

Preface

First, I would like to thank all patients who shared their personal stories with CRPS in this book. We recently published the first volume, which included the stories of several patients who live suffering from CRPS. When we talk about suffering, it is not only pain, but suffering made some patients commit suicide or have an amputation to get rid of the pain.

CRPS is a very serious condition and dealing with it otherwise is not wise. Unfortunately, there is a huge lack of knowledge even among health care providers about the seriousness of this condition and what it can lead to if not managed quickly and aggressively. Early and aggressive management can lead to control and even cure of the pain, but lack of diagnosis and not understanding the urgency of treating this condition can lead to a worsening of pain with associated depression, anxiety, limb atrophy, amputation, and potential suicide.

My friend Eric and I authored volumes I and II of this book to share the stories of patients suffering from CRPS. Our goal is to increase public awareness of the severity of this condition. What we mean by the public is everyone from employers, spouses, health care providers, and others. It is very important to provide support to CRPS patients to avoid the serious consequences of the condition. Employers should understand the limitations of their employees; "yes, the condition can cause pain to touch," spouses need to support their partners with CRPS, and health care providers should treat it aggressively and quickly. If they have limited experience treating this condition, then they should immediately refer the patient to the experts.

With CRPS, we are racing against time, and providers should start with a non-pharmacological treatment, then medications, and if they fail, then interventions. If one modality is not working, health care providers should move to the next modality without waiting. They should discuss a plan with the patient, with one step after another, and this depends on the success or failure of different modalities.

I hope this book will help increase public awareness about the condition and help CRPS patients to understand the seriousness of this condition and the need to seek help as soon as possible without waiting for too long.

Alaa Abd-Elsayed, MD, MPH, FASA

Preface

I would like to especially thank all the CRPS patients for taking the time to write and share their stories. It is generous of all of you to share your journey of living with this painful disease in this book. Your willingness to share your story will provide great help and support to others who are suffering from CRPS.

I have been working in the CRPS community for over 32 years to help advocate for other CRPS patients. As, being a sufferer of CRPS for over 35 years, and being an amputee for 12 years, I understand the struggles and pain that CRPS patients endure. The biggest downfall for most patients is the lack of understanding of CRPS by the medical community and the public.

I have been fortunate to know and work with my friend Doctor Alaa Abd-Elsayed over the years. It has been a great honor for me to work on this fourth book with Doctor Al and all the patients that were so gracious enough to submit their stories.

2

We both felt that writing this book that shared patient's personal stories of living life as an Amputee with CRPS would help to continue spreading the desperately needed awareness, help educate the public and the medical community that CRPS is a real and serious disease.

I hope this book will be helpful and provide reassurance to other CRPS patients that they are not alone; with their daily battle of dealing with the chronic pain of CRPS and coping with being an amputee as well. Moreover, I also hope this book will help the medical community worldwide to understand how patients live and cope with this unrelenting painful disease. Remember we all have to work together to help spread awareness in finding a cure for CRPS.

Eric M. Phillips

INTRODUCTION

Alaa Abd-Elsayed, MD, MPH, FASA, and Eric M. Phillips

Complex regional pain syndrome (CRPS), is a poorly understood condition by the medical community. Many patients may suffer long before getting diagnosed or even receive proper treatment.

CRPS is a painful disease that affects the patient physically, mentally, and emotionally. To obtain a complete understanding of this disease, one must read the patient's personal story to get a sense of what can potentially happen to some patients.

The purpose of this book is to share the stories of CRPS patients that have reached the end-stage of the disease, and had to have an amputation due to many issues such as infection or the loss of use of the limb. These amputations were only done to help save the patient's life and give them a better quality of life.

As we are all well aware of CRPS is a complex disease to diagnose, treat, and to understand. Treating physicians must take into consideration that each patient is affected differently by CRPS due to the different stages of the disease. The patient and treating physician need to work as a team to create a proper treatment plan that will help the patient control their pain.

CRPS has become a global disease, with millions of cases worldwide. CRPS affects patients in the same way. It does not matter if the patient lives in the United States, Australia, Britain, France or anywhere else in the world. Every CRPS patient suffers from the same chronic pain and has difficulty in receiving proper treatment. Unfortunately, CRPS patients must fight daily to deal with their pain and try to get the recognition that CRPS is an actual disease.

We have created this book to help share how patients suffer from the pain of CRPS. Until a doctor, relative, or friend sees the damage that CRPS causes, one cannot comprehend the pain patients deal with daily. These stories you will read in this book range from patients having early stages of the disease to the end-stage of the disease.

We understand how debilitating CRPS is for patients and how difficult it is for a patient to make the choice of having an amputation when they have reached the end-stage of the disease.

Please remember, the purpose of this book is not to advocate amputation, we simply are sharing the stories of CRPS patients who have had amputations. Having an amputation should only be reserved for patients in end-stages of the disease. It should not be considered a treatment option.

Our main goal for this book is to help spread awareness about CRPS. Educating the medical community on the topic of CRPS is a high priority. The medical community needs to understand how devastating CRPS is and how it affects the patient physically, mentally, and emotionally.

COMPLEX REGIONAL PAIN SYNDROME (CRPS),

AMPUTATION, and PHANTOM PAIN

Eric M. Phillips

International RSD Foundation

www.rsdinfo.com

Abstract: For centuries, the great pioneers in the medical community (past and present) from around the world have written about complex regional pain syndrome (CRPS), amputation, and phantom pain. CRPS is known as one of the most painful conditions a person can endure. In a small population of CRPS patients who have endured many forms of failed treatments, and reached the end-stage of the disease, the only option for most of these patients is to amputate the affected limb, to help save their lives and give them a better quality of life. Amputation should not be the first option of treatment for CRPS patients, because of the many side effects of having the surgery such as phantom pain, infections, and spread of CRPS, which are just a few examples of what patients may face doing this surgery. In this chapter, I will discuss the effects of CRPS, amputation, and phantom pain.

Keywords: Causalgia, complex regional pain syndrome (CRPS), reflex sympathetic dystrophy (RSD), amputation, phantoms, phantom limb, phantom pain, phantom sensation.

HISTORY OF CRPS

Complex regional pain syndrome (CRPS) also known as reflex sympathetic dystrophy (RSD), and causalgia have been documented around the world for centuries. Ambroise Paré was one of the first to describe what is now called CRPS, through his account of the persistent pain that King Charles IX had suffered from in the 16th century (1,2). In the late 1700's British surgeon Sir Pervcivall Pott recognized burning pain and atrophy in injured extremities (2-4). In 1813, Denmark reported a single case of a soldier who had an amputation due to burning pain (2,3,5,6). In 1838 Hamilton had seen some cases in which his patients had symptoms of what we call causalgia that resulted from accidental nerve injuries (2,7). Early in 1864 Paget had patients who had symptoms of constant warmth in their limbs after nerve injury (2,8). Also, in 1864, Silas Weir Mitchell the father of American neurology gave the description of causalgia in his classic article Gunshot Wounds and Other Injuries of Nerves, but it was not until 1867 when he coined the term of causalgia from the Greek words, "Kausos" (heat) and "algos" (pain) to describe this syndrome (2,9). Mitchell was the first to describe of this painful syndrome in the United States. Some of the symptoms that his patients suffering from causalgia had been burning pain and glossy skin. He mentioned that the burning pain came first and the skin changes came afterward. *To quote Mitchell, he stated that "Causalgia is the most terrible of all the tortures a nerve wound may inflict."*

Over the past centuries, these medical pioneers have opened the window to one of the most puzzling and painful conditions that a person can suffer from.

Complex Regional Pain Syndrome (CRPS)

Complex regional pain syndrome (CRPS) is a painful condition that can be caused by minor trauma or surgery. There are two types of pain that a patient may experience with CRPS. The burning pain, the feeling that their limb is on fire, or the ice-cold pain feeling of their limb is immersed in a bucket of ice. The pain of CRPS is felt 24-hours a day, seven days a week, and the pain of CRPS never lets up for a majority of these patients.

During the course of the disease, most CRPS patients endure multiple treatments and procedures to try to obtain some form of pain relief. A majority of these procedures and treatments fail and may cause the spread of the disease.

Treatments from nerve blocks, medications, surgical procedures such as sympathectomy (surgical, chemical, or radiofrequency), spinal cord stimulator (SCS), or infusion pump have failed or spread CRPS in some patients.

CRPS can cause some of the following symptoms:

- Burning pain in the extremities
- Chronic pain after injury or surgery
- Cold feeling in the extremities
- Discoloration of the skin
- Edema (Swelling of the extremities)
- Hypersensitivity to touch
- Limited range of motion
- Muscle spasms

CRPS can affect the upper extremities, lower extremities, there have been reported cases of facial CRPS, internal organ involvement, and cases of total body CRPS.

According to my mentor the late Doctor Hooshmand, there are four stages of the disease (2,3). These stages may come and go during the course of the patient's CRPS. Below are the four stages of CRPS:

- Stage I: Dysfunction
- Stage II: Dystrophy

- Stage III: Atrophy
- Stage IV: Irreversible disturbance of plasticity; autonomic failure.

It is well known that during the long duration of the disease when patients reach stage IV, they start to develop various complications such as disturbance of the immune system (neurogenic inflammation), limbic system, cardiac system, endocrine system, and respiratory system. These are just a few of the various complications of CRPS (2,10,11). These complications are not recognized by the medical community. The medical community must understand that these complications are real and that patients do suffer from these various complications of CRPS.

History of Amputation

Amputations have been performed for centuries worldwide. In 1552, Ambroise Paré was one of the first military surgeons to use amputation for the treatment of gunshot wounds and infections during the wars in Europe (12). He was the first to choose the site of amputation on a patient. He also performed amputations above the gangrenous area of the affected limb (12). In 1554, Ambroise Paré designed an artificial wooden limb for his amputee patients. These artificial limbs were functional with moving joints. He used springs and metal gears to help with the aid of gripping for the fingers and he also made artificial legs (13). In his work with his amputee patients, he did mention some patients suffering from phantom limb, this was around 1545, but he did not write about the phantom limb until 1552 (13,14). Ambroise Paré was ahead of his time with his work with performing amputations and designing artificial limbs. He is also known as the Father of modern prosthetics.

Silas Weir Mitchell the Father of American Neurology was another pioneer in the field of amputation during the American Civil War. During the Civil

War, he was asked by his friend William Hammond the Surgeon General for the Union to work at the Turner Lane Hospital (also known as "Stump Hospital") in Philadelphia, PA. While working at the hospital with the help of his colleagues George Morehouse and William W. Keen, he treated a large group of soldiers who were injured during the war (15,16). These soldiers had nerve injuries and amputations. Through Mitchell's work during the Civil War, he coined the term Causalgia which is now known as complex regional pain syndrome (CRPS), and he also coined the term Phantom pain, which his patients suffered from after having an amputation due to their injuries from the war. I will discuss more on Mitchell's work on phantom pain later in this chapter.

Silas Weir Mitchell was also ahead of his time with his contributions to the field of Neurology. His work with soldiers wounded in battle, where he recognized the burning pain and phantom pain that these soldiers were suffering from. His work and research into Causalgia and phantom pain has been helpful to doctors in the present day to help patients now suffering from CRPS and who have had amputations.

During the Civil War, there were 30,000 limbs amputated due to war injuries. Mitchell reported that the patient's stumps have become extremely sensitive after amputation. Also, these patients developed Chorea (a movement disorder that caused involuntary muscle movement in the stump). He also reported the use of ice was too painful for the patients to use (16).

CRPS and Amputation

CRPS and amputations have been documented for centuries by many pioneers of medicine from Ambroise Paré to Silas Weir Mitchell and beyond. One must remember that a majority of these amputations were performed during wartime due to the injuries that the soldiers sustained during battle.

The use of amputation in the treatment of CRPS is not the first option in the management of the disease. Amputation should only be used in end-stages cases of the disease when all other treatments have failed. Even when most forms of treatments have failed, the patients and their treating physicians should not jump into the idea of having an amputation. Doing an amputation when one has CRPS should only be done when the patient is in the end-stage of the disease and when the disease affects the patient's health due to infection, loss of use of the limb, or other side-effects that may be caused by CRPS. When patients come to the point where having an amputation may be their only option to help save their life and give them a better quality of life, it should be considered, but many things should be taken into consideration before the final decision is made.

From my personal experience of having CRPS for 35 years and being an amputee for 12 years, I recommend to all patients that, they should think long and hard before doing an amputation when suffering from CRPS. I inform patients that they cannot wake up one day and say hey, I want to amputate my limb. Doing an amputation is a big altering change in a person's life. I recommend that patients who are considering having an amputation, make an appointment with a good pain Psychologist who understands CRPS. Seeing a Psychologist helped me in making my decision of having an amputation done. The other helpful thing is to have a good surgeon who will take the time to answer your questions that you may have regarding having the surgery and to talk about your hopes and fears about having an amputation. The other thing that is helpful, is to find a good prosthetist who will take the time to inform you about what options you have when the time comes to be fitted for your new prosthetic after your surgery and to answers any questions and concerns that you may have about wearing a prosthesis. Also, talking with your family and friend is very helpful too. It helps them know and understand what you are doing and what you will be going through. You never want to shock someone you know that you had an amputation because you never told them. So, there are many things to take into consideration before having an amputation done. Remember amputation is not a cure-all for CRPS.

Over the centuries and decades, there have been many case studies of CRPS patients having amputations. This is not a new approach in the treatment of CRPS. One should not consider amputation as a form of treatment for CRPS. Amputation is a result of an end-stage case of the disease when all other forms of treatments have failed and the patient's health is at risk.

Case Reports

In 1813, Surgeon Alexander Denmark reported a single case of a soldier who had an amputation at the elbow due to burning pain in their arm. (2,3,5,6).

In 1916, René Leriche, during World War I, saw more than 30 cases of amputation in which neurectomies were performed. None of these patients were cured by the procedure. He found the use of Novocain infiltrations into the paravertebral sympathetic chain, provided a new and effective method for giving relief to his patients (17).

In 1987, Rohrich, et al., reported on a case of end-stage CRPS in a 34-year-old female who sustained minor trauma to her left thumb. She suffered from CRPS for 21 years. The patient was untreated for many years. Her hand became painful and deformed. Unfortunately, this patient had to have her left hand amputated. Rohrich, et al, states that this case presents an example of the importance of early diagnosis and treatment of CRPS to prevent patients from having an amputation (18).

In 1992, Erdmann and Wynn-Jones reviewed two cases of CRPS from the same family who underwent amputations four years apart. Both cases had above-elbow amputations. (19).

In 1993, Veldmand, et al., have reported 19 patients with chronic lymphedema due to CRPS. The chronic relapsing infections were resistant to treatment. They reported that five patients in their study required amputation (2,20).

In 1995, Dielissen and colleagues reported the results of amputation in 28 CRPS patients who had undergone 34 amputations in 31 limbs (2,21).

- Three patients had two limbs amputated and three patients had two amputations performed on one limb.

- In 28 patients they had recurrent CRPS in the residual limb(stump).

- In 29 out of 34 amputations performed developed phantom sensation and 24 cases developed phantom pain.

- Twenty-two patients were fitted for prostheses and only two could use the prosthetic. The other 20 cases could not use the prostheses due to recurring CRPS in the stump.

- Five patients had recurring infections.

- Two patients had their symptoms of CRPS reversed from the surgery.

In their conclusion, Dielissen and colleagues believe that for patients with severe chronic CRPS, amputation should not be performed due to pain alone. They found that amputation done in cases with severe incurable infections was more successful and they feel that the amputation should be performed at a level where the patient does not have any signs and symptoms of CRPS. They report that after amputation for patients with CRPS, they are unlikely to wear a prosthesis (21).

In 1997, Geertzen, et al., reported a 26-year-old female who after three and a half years had undergone an amputation of the left-hand due to recurring infection. According to Geertzen and his group, amputation should only be performed when a patient has irreversible changes that cause loss of function of the limb and intolerable chronic pain caused by the CRPS (22).

In 1998, van der Laan, et al., reviewed 1,006 RSD-CRPS cases. They reported that 13 out of 30 had infected CRPS extremities, and these patients had a subsequent amputation. In their group of patients showed skin lesions only had skin ulcers. Also, in their study, they make a valid point that patients with "cold-CRPS" vs. "warm-CRPS" have a higher risk for developing severe complications from the disease (23). This should be taken into consideration when evaluating CRPS patients for any type of treatment.

In 1999, Hooshmand and Hashmi wrote a review of 824 CRPS cases. In their review, they reported 11 patients who had undergone amputation due to infections and severe edema. In all 11 patients, they showed marked deterioration postoperatively. The stump became a new source of CRPS in these patients. In 2008, they had their twelfth CRPS patient who underwent amputation due to long-lasting infections (that patient was me). Out of the twelve patients, only one was able to wear a prosthetic (once again that patient was me). Doctor Hooshmand stated that amputation should be avoided by all means due to its side effects of aggravation of pain and the tendency for the spread of CRPS (2,24).

In 2016, Midbair, et al., authored an article regarding amputation in patients with CRPS: a comparative study between amputees and non-amputees. In their study, they reviewed two groups that had a total of 19 patients in each group. These groups consisted of non-amputated CRPS patients and amputated CRPS patients. The amputated group showed better results compared to the non-amputated group. They suggest that amputation should be saved for patients with end-stage CRPS (25).

In 2020, Geertzen, et al, published a review on a 15-year study that was performed from May 2000 to September 2015, which was conducted at the University Medical Center Groningen in the Netherlands. This was a study of the outcome of amputations performed on CRPS patients (26).

In their 15-year study, they documented 53 CRPS patients undergoing amputation at their hospital. Only 48 patients participated in the study (26).

- Thirty-seven patients showed improvement in their mobility.

- Thirty- five patients had a reduction of pain after amputation.

- One patient had a recurrence of CRPS in their residual limb and three patients had a recurrence of CRPS in another limb.

- Thirty-five patients were fitted for a prosthesis for their lower limbs. Only 24 patients were still using their prosthesis at the end of the study.

All these amputations were performed due to unbearable chronic pain, life-threatening infections, or the loss of use of the affected limb due to CRPS (26).

In their conclusion, Geertzen, et al., stated that amputation for CRPS may be considered as a form of treatment for end-stage cases of CRPS (26).

These case studies of CRPS and amputation are just a few examples of the many published reports on this subject. As, we know, the subject of CRPS and amputations has been documented for centuries and decades. More research by the medical community is needed into this option of treatment for end-stage CRPS cases.

History of Phantom Pain

Phantom pain has been documented for centuries from around the world. Throughout history phantom pain has been documented by many of the pioneers of medicine, Paré, Mitchell, Bell, Müller, and many of today's great researchers. Phantom pain has been an enigma to many in the medical field for centuries. The work by these pioneers has helped place a name on this phenomenon we call Phantom pain.

The earliest mention of symtoms of phantom pain was reported by Ambroise Paré in 1552, René Descartes in 1637, Aaron Lemos in 1798, Charles Bell in 1811, Johannes Müller in 1834, and by Silas Weir Mitchell in 1871(13,14,16,27-32).

Phantom Pain

Phantom pain is one of the most torturous pain anyone can suffer after having an amputation. It is one of the most relentless pains other than the pain of CRPS a person could ever suffer from.

In 1545, Ambroise Paré did experience working with amputee patients who had symptoms of phantom sensations-phantom limb pain, but he did not write about it until 1552 (13,27).

In 1637, René Descartes had written about phantom sensations. He had a theory that the sensations his patients felt involved the machinery of the brain (13,28).

In 1798, Aaron Lemos saw three cases of phantom limbs and he wrote his dissertation on phantom limbs. The title of his dissertation was: *The Continuing Pain of an Amputated Limb.* He mentions in his dissertation the following: *There are amputees who, a long time after undergoing the operation, complaining of severe pain precisely at the place where the affected part had been previously been troublesome* (13,29).

In 1811, Charles Bell reported that stimulating the nerves in the stump of amputees can cause a sensation that feels like it was coming from the missing extremity, which he felt provided clear evidence that there was brain involvement in these cases (13,30).

In 1834, Johannes Müller followed six cases of phantom limb. He had followed these patients for 12 years and longer. He also felt that patients with phantom limbs were unlikely to undergo remission of this pain. To quote Müller: *"The belief that these sensations are lost a short time after amputation is an error of medical men, who generally do not watch the*

17

patients longer than a few hours". Another important fact that Müller recognized, was the change of weather can affect phantoms (13,31).

In 1871, Silas Weir Mitchell during the American civil war, is where he coined the term Phantom pain from his work with soldiers that lost their limbs during the battles of the civil war (13,32).

During Mitchell's time working as a neurologist in the American civil war he saw so much suffering that the soldiers had sustained from their injuries on the battlefield. These soldiers developed causalgia (now known as CRPS) and had amputations due to limb injuries. This has made him a pioneer in causalgia-CRPS, amputation, and phantom pain.

In his book titled: Injuries of Nerves and Their Consequences (16), Mitchell wrote:

"Nearly every man who loses a limb carries about with him a constant or inconstant phantom of the missing member, a sensory ghost of that much of himself, and sometimes a most inconvenient presence, faintly felt at times, but ready to be called up to his perception by a blow, a touch, or a change of wind." This is a great observation that every amputee goes through (16).

Also, in his book Mitchell wrote, that eighty-six out of ninety amputees had sensory phantom sensations. He also stated that the amputated limb is rarely felt as a whole when the patient has phantom pain. It is nearly the foot or the hand, the toes or the fingers that are recognized by the patient (16).

He also discussed in his writings that patients suffering from phantom pain can sense weather changes, which he found puzzling. He also noted the differences between arm and leg phantoms, and how ghost sensations may be affected by an artificial limb (16).

Mitchell, was troubled that there were no effective ways to treat the painful phantom pain, even after performing additional amputations, cauterization, acupuncture, nerve resections, and many other forms of treatments including using opiates, which all short-lived for pain relief for these patients. He was also the first to report using a local injection of morphine to treat phantom pain (13,16).

Mitchell's pioneer work with causalgia, amputation, and phantom pain, should be recognized as a great contribution to modern medicine. We can continue to learn from his research work. He has left a lot of answers to these complicated pains in his writings.

CRPS, Amputation, Phantom Pain - "A Patients Perspective"

As I have mentioned earlier in this chapter; I have suffered from CRPS for 35 years, and I have been an amputee for the past 12 years, and I have suffered from phantom pain since having my amputation. Having CRPS is a difficult disease to live with and to treat. Getting a diagnosis may take time for some patients (as in my case it took two-and-a-half years to receive my diagnosis). In most cases, treatment and surgery seem to fail, and it may also cause the spread of the disease as in my case, and for a majority of patients.

After years of failed treatments, and surgery that made my CRPS spread up my leg past my knee, I spent years with the loss of uses of my left leg. For over 20 years I lived having a useless limb that I had to deal with the unrelenting pain of CRPS and when I reached the end-stage of the disease I had to battle infections in my foot and leg for over a year and a half. After many rounds of oral and I.V. antibiotics and numerous stays at the hospital to try to control the infections, all the treatments failed to help control the infections. I was at the point where nothing was helping the infections and I was running out of options. During my last stay in the hospital to treat these infections, my doctors had a discussion with me about amputation. This was a discussion I never wanted to hear, but I always knew in the back of my mind that this might be an option for me someday in the future. I also said to myself and my family, that I would only do an amputation if the CRPS affected my health (such as infection). Well, in my twenty-third year of having CRPS, I was at that point that the disease and the infections were affecting my health. My doctors told me that if I did not do the amputation, and stayed on the same path trying to treat the infections, that I would be dead within five to six months.

So, trying to decide to have an amputation is a big pill to swallow. It is a big decision to make in life. It took a month to make my decision to have the amputation. I had done my research for some time on the effects of having an amputation with CRPS. I was fortunate to have a great vascular surgeon, who listen to me about my hopes and fears of having this surgery. I think it's important that the surgeon and patient take the time to discuss the many pros and cons of having an amputation with CRPS. I feel that the patient, surgeon, and the whole medical team have to be on the same page. Having an amputation is a major decision to make and a life-changing event in one's life.

One aspect that helped me in making my decision to have the amputation, was to speak with a Psychologist, who put things in the best perspective for me. She asked me if my leg was my friend or the enemy at this time in my life? I said to her that it was my enemy. After that discussion, I made my decision to have the surgery. I was at the point that the infections were not getting better nor was the pain from the CRPS getting any better either. I was only sleeping one to two hours a night due to the severe pain from the CRPS and the infections. Well, I had made my decision to have the amputation after speaking with my family and friends.

A week before my surgery, I had met with my vascular surgeon, to review our plan of doing the surgery. Once my surgeon saw how bad the infections had gotten, he said he had to rethink his plan of action for the surgery. He decided to perform a two-stage amputation. He recommended the first day of surgery, we should amputate the foot at the ankle, so that we could let the rest of the infection drain out of my leg before performing the second stage of the surgery an above-knee amputation. At, this point of hearing his strategies for my surgery, I had agreed to use his plan.

In regards, to the level of amputation, I recommended to my surgeon, that we go above the line of discoloration that I had on my leg due to the CRPS. My surgeon agreed with me on this decision. Looking at the history of the work done by Ambroise Paré who was one of the first military surgeons to use amputation for the treatment of gunshot wounds and infections (12,14). He was also the first to choose the site of amputation on a patient. He also performed amputations above the gangrenous area of the affected limb (12,14). I feel that this is an important way to approach the idea of performing an amputation on CRPS patients. By going past this line of discoloration due to CRPS, it may help with eliminating the potential spread of CRPS in the residual limb? In my case, I did not have any spread of the disease. This option should be taken into consideration for both the patient and surgeon. In my case, I am grateful that my surgeon, listen to my request of doing the amputation at this level. I have been told by both my surgeon and prosthetist that I made the right decision.

Another factor with performing an amputation in CRPS cases is the potential of spread of the disease. In my case, I followed my mentor the late Doctor Hooshmand's protocol of doing an epidural nerve block (containing Marcaine and Depo-Medrol®) around the clock while I was in the hospital to help prevent the spread of CRPS in the residual limb. By doing this method, it did help prevent any spread of the disease.

After my amputation surgery, I faced a long road of rehabilitation, to gain my strength back and to work on getting my stump into shape to get ready to be fitter for my first prosthetic socket. I spent about two years in physical therapy to learn how to walk on my prosthetic leg. It was not easy for me since I had not walked on two legs in over 20 years. I have to be honest it is not easy walking on a prosthetic when you have a short limb. But I have done it, with the help of my great team of doctors, prosthetists, and physical therapists.

At, the time of my amputation I had lived 23 years with CRPS. Living with the pain of CRPS is one I would never want to wish on anyone. It is an awful pain that never stops. But, after my amputation, I was introduced to phantom pain. In my personal opinion, I feel that phantom pain is the most brutal type of pain one can endure. I feel that phantom pain is worse than CRPS pain. Again, this is just my personal opinion.

I am aware that some amputees have never endured phantom pain. But, in my case, I have had phantom pain since my surgery. Phantom pain is a strange phenomenon at times. It can come and go anytime it likes and it never gives you a warning. In my case few days before a storm is coming in, I start to have phantom pain, it can happen at any time during the day or night. In my research about phantom pain, I was amazed to read that both Doctors Johannes Müller and Silas Weir Mitchell reported that their patient's phantom pain was also affected by weather changes.

Over the years, there has been much debate about phantom pain and phantom sensations. In my personal experience, they are both the same. When I get the "so-called" phantom sensations, they are still painful. So why classify it just as a sensation? To me pain is pain. Phantom pain or phantom sensations are all the same. They are both painful!

When a patient has phantom pain or phantom sensations it should not be discounted. They both cause a form of pain. Phantom pain just lasts longer than a phantom sensation. Phantom pain can last for hours to days vs. phantom sensation can last a few seconds to a few minutes.

The phenomenon of phantom pain or phantom sensations is not in the patient's head. It is real. The unfortunate thing is most treatments either injections or oral medications do not help control this type of pain.

As the years have gone by and living life with both CRPS and being an amputee, I know that phantom pain is just part of my life living as an amputee. When I get phantom pain, it feels like I am being repeatedly stabbed over and over. This can go on for hours to days for me.

I have found a strange thing about phantom pain that it changes locations on my foot and leg every time. Sometimes it will attack my last three toes, then there are times I feel it in just my great toe, and then there are times I feel it on the bottom of my foot or in other parts of my leg. I have never felt my leg as a whole. You would think that since the leg is no longer there, that I would feel the leg as a whole and just not certain sections of my foot and toes.

According to Doctor Mitchell's research on phantom pain, he stated that the limb is rarely felt as a whole. Most patients just feel the foot or hand, or just the toes and fingers. I can attest to his observations.

In 12 years of being an amputee, I have only felt phantom pain in my knee six-times. The other things I have felt when I have had phantom pain are the areas where I had my infections, the screw that was in my great toe, and where they did the first amputation at my ankle.

A prosthetics is the biggest life-line for an amputee. In some cases of CRPS patients who have undergone an amputation due to infections and end-stages of the disease, unfortunately, cannot wear a prosthesis due to many factors such as pain or sensitivity in their stumps or for other reasons.

I am fortunate that I can use a prosthesis. One of the first lessons that I had learned from my prosthetist was that you must have a proper fit with your prosthetic socket. If the socket is not fitting properly, the prosthesis will be useless to the patient. I have been fortunate to work with some great prosthetist, and over the years, and I have met many amputees who could not wear their prosthesis, because of a poorly fitting prosthetic socket, so it is important to find a prosthetist that will make you a good fitting prosthetic socket. I also tell other amputees that if their socket is not fitting properly or it causes them pain or discomfort, to call their prosthetist right away so they can make adjustments to it so it will be comfortable for you to wear and use. Remember, they want you to call them if you have an issue. They are there to help you and they want you up and walking.

There are many factors that patients and their medical team should take into consideration when the subject of amputation is considered as a treatment option for end-stage cases of the disease. The number one thing is to have open discussions about all the pros and cons of amputation with your surgeon and family.

Here is a list of recommendations patients should consider while deciding to have an amputation:

- Review the pros and cons of having an amputation.

- Consult with a surgeon who understands CRPS.

- Consult with a Psychologist who works with pain patients.

- Consult with a knowledgeable prosthetist to discuss prosthetic options either before or after the amputation.

- Consult with a physical therapist who has worked with both CRPS and amputee patients.

- Speak with other CRPS patients who have had an amputation.

These are all important things patients should have on their checklist when they are making the biggest decision of their life to have an amputation. Patients have to remember that they are the CEO of their health care and life. Patients have to be surrounded by doctors, Psychologist, prosthetist, and physical therapist who they have confidence in when it comes to their health care. All patients need to have a team that will support them in making this life-changing decision.

In my case, I feel that having the amputation was a success for many reasons. It helped save my life, it controlled the infections that I had suffered from, it has allowed me to walk again, and it has given me a better quality of life.

Research

Research is vital when it comes to dealing with CRPS. When adding amputation into the mix with CRPS, we need to accumulate as much data as possible to help physicians and patients make the right decision when a patient reaches the end-stage of CRPS and there is no other option left for them, other than having an amputation.

The research and case studies done by the Dutch group of Doctors Dielissen, Geertzen, Goris, Veldman, and van der Laan, have been most helpful in showing the results of amputation in the CRPS population.

We need to continue with researching the effects that amputation has on CRPS patients. Reports of the pros and cons of this surgery can be useful when a patient is deciding to have an amputation for end-stage CRPS.

Conclusion

For hundreds of years, there have been many documented cases of CRPS, amputation, and phantom pain worldwide. CRPS is a disease that is difficult for many physicians to understand and treat. CRPS is a painful disease for patients to live with. When patients reach the end-stage of the disease, it leaves them with few options. Because of complications such as loss of use of the limb and infections, amputation may be the only option for these patients.

There has been much debate over the years when a CRPS patient should have an amputation? It's a great question to ask. How far into the disease should it be before an amputation should be considered? For example, I recall a case while I was working with my mentor the late Doctor Hooshmand. We saw a case in his clinic where the patient had end-stage

CRPS in their right hand and arm. Over time the neuro-inflammation and the infections became so severe that the only option for this patient was to have an amputation (the patient's hand was so swollen that it looks like a Boxer's Glove). The unfortunate thing is this patient went to see multiple surgeons and no one would perform an amputation. It took years before this patient was able to find a surgeon who was willing to do the amputation, which did help save this patient's life and gave this patient a better quality of life after surgery.

Was it fair for this patient to be put through years of torture and pain because a few doctors would not operate and do an amputation for this patient? Looking back at this case the answer is NO it was not fair! This patient should not have had to wait years for the amputation. It was clear that she had an end-stage case of CRPS due to the severe and grossly swollen and infected hand and arm that was affecting her health and her quality of life. No one should have to suffer as this patient did. These doctors did a disservice to this patient and caused many years of unnecessary suffering. In this case, amputation was the best option for this patient.

Remember, having an amputation is not a cure-all for CRPS. It may cause other complications such as phantom pain, infections, the spread of CRPS, and not being able to wear a prosthesis.

Amputation should only be entertained when a patient has developed incurable infection, or has reached the end-stage of the disease (which includes the loss of use of the limb).

Patients must understand all the pros and cons of undergoing this life-changing surgery. They need to research every aspect of the issues that may arise from having the surgery, and find the right medical team to work with. The number one thing is patients need to be mentally prepared to have an amputation and be able to adjust to life living as an amputee with CRPS. From personal experience, it's not an easy thing to deal with at times.

There can be some significant benefits for patients undergoing amputation for end-stage CRPS, and there can be some disastrous results for some patients after amputation. There have been some patients who are fortunate to become pain free after amputation.

After amputation, the physician, patient, physical therapist, and prosthetist cannot jump the gun and rush the healing process. CRPS patients who have undergone amputation have to take extra precautions and allow the stump to heal properly to avoid any issues such as infections, open wounds, and spread of CRPS. Having CRPS can add a twist to things such as healing and wearing a prothesis for some patients. Do not rush the healing process. This will help the patient in the long run.

I wrote this chapter not to advocate or promote amputation for CRPS patients. I wrote it to inform patients about the history of CRPS, amputation, phantom pain and to share the history and some case studies about this difficult topic of amputation and CRPS.

We need more research into the effects of amputation in CRPS cases. It's important that physicians and patients work together to help understand the effects of amputation on such issues as the spread of CRPS, and phantom pain. It's vital that we have more research and data to help guide the physicians and patients when the only option for patients with end-stage CRPS is amputation.

References

1. Paré A. Les Ouvres d' Ambroise Paré, King Charles IX. 10th Book, Chapter 41. Paris Gabriel Buon 1598 : 401.

2. Hooshmand H, Phillips EM. Various Complications of Complex Regional Pain Syndrome (CRPS). Neurological Associates Pain Management Center, Vero Beach, Florida. www.rsdinfo.com and www.rsdrx.com Feb 16, 2016

3. Hooshmand H. Chronic Pain: Reflex Sympathetic Dystrophy: Prevention and Management. CRC Press, Boca Raton FL. 1993.

4. Casten DF, Betcher AM. Reflex sympathetic dystrophy. Surg Gynecol Obstet 1955; 100: 97–101.

5. Denmark A. An example of symptoms resembling tic douloureux produced by a wound in the radial nerve. Med Chir Trans 1819; 4:48.

6. Richards RL. Causalgia: a centennial review. Arch Neurol 1967; 16:339.

7. Hamilton, J. On some effects resulting from wounds of nerves. Dublin J Med Sc 1838; 13: 38–55.

8. Paget J. Clinical lecture on some cases of local paralysis. Med Times Hosp Gaz 1864; 1:331.

9. Mitchell SW, Morehouse GR, Keen WW. Gunshot wounds and other injuries of nerves. Philadelphia: Lippincott, 1864.

10. Hooshmand, H, Hashmi, M, Phillips, EM. Venipuncture Complex Regional Pain Syndrome Type II. American Journal of Pain Management October 2001; 11: 112-124. http://www.rsdinfo.com/Venipuncture_CRPS-II_Article.pdf

11. Phillips EM: The Misconceptions of Complex Regional Pain Syndrome (CRPS). In: Complex Regional Pain Syndrome (CRPS): Patients' Perspective of Living in Chronic Pain. Volume II. MG Academy, LLC Publisher. July 2020, Pgs 6-34.

12. Hernigou P. Ambroise Paré II: Paré's contributions to amputation and ligature. Int Orthop. 2013 Apr;37(4):769-772.

13. Finger S, Hustwit MP. Five early accounts of phantom limb in context: Paré, Descartes, Lemos, Bell, and Mitchell. Neurosurgery 2003 ; 52(3) :675-686.

14. Paré A. *La Méthode de Traicter les Playes Faictes par Hacquebutes et Aultres Bastons à Feu.* Paris, Chés Viuant Gaulterot, 1545.

15. Kline DG. Silas Weir Mitchell and "The Strange Case of George Dedlow". Neurosurg Focus. 2016; 41: 1-7.

16. Mitchell SW: *Injuries of Nerves and Their Consequences* Philadelphia, JB Lippincott, 1872.

17. Leriche R., La Chirurgie de la Douleur. Paris : Masson, 1937.

18. Rohrich, RJ, Stevenson, TR, Piepgrass, W, et al: End-Stage Reflex Sympathetic Dystrophy, Plastic and Reconstructive Surgery 1987; 79 (4): 625-626.

19. Erdmann MW, Wynn-Jones CH. 'Familial' reflex sympathetic dystrophy syndrome and amputation. Injury. 1992;23(2):136-138.

20. Veldman PH, Reynen HM, Arntz IE, et al. Signs and symptoms of reflex sympathetic dystrophy: prospective study of 829 patients. Lancet 1993; 342:1012-1016. http://www.ncbi.nlm.nih.gov/pubmed/8105263

21. Dielissen PW, Claassen AT, Veldman PH, Goris RJ. Amputation for reflex sympathetic dystrophy. J Bone Joint Surg Br. 1995; 77(2):270-273. PMID: 7706345.

22. Geertzen JH, Rietman JS, Smit AJ, et al. A young female patient with reflex sympathetic dystrophy of the upper limb in whom amputation became inevitable. Prosthet Orthot Int. 1997;21(2):159-161. doi: 10.3109/03093649709164545. PMID: 9285961.

23. van der Laan L, Veldman PH, Goris RJ. Severe complications of reflex sympathetic dystrophy: infection, ulcers, chronic edema, dystonia, and myoclonus. Arch Phys Med Rehabil. 1998;79(4):424-429. doi: 10.1016/s0003-9993(98)90144-7. PMID: 9552109.

24. Hooshmand H, and Hashmi. Complex regional pain syndrome (CRPS, RSDS) diagnosis and therapy. A review of 824 patients. Pain Digest 1999; 9: 1-24.

25. Midbari A, Suzan E, Adler T, et al. Amputation in patients with complex regional pain syndrome: a comparative study between amputees and non-amputees with intractable disease. Bone Joint J. 2016;98-B (4):548-554. doi: 10.1302/0301-620X.98B4.36422. PMID: 27037439.

26. Geertzen JHB, Scheper J, Schrier E, Dijkstra PU. Outcomes of amputation due to long-standing therapy-resistant complex regional pain syndrome type I. J Rehabil Med. 2020; 24;52(8): jrm00087. doi: 10.2340/16501977-2718. PMID: 32735019.

27. Paré A. La Manière de Traicter les Playes Faictes tant par Hacquebutes que par flèches. Paris, Iean de Brie, 1551.

28. Descartes R: The Philosophical Writings of Descartes, Vol. 3: The Correspondence. Cottingham J, Stoothoff R, Murdoch D, Kenny A (trans). New York, Cambridge University Press, 1991.

29. Lemos A: Dolorem membri amputati remanentem explicat: Dissertatio Inauguralis Medica. Halae. In Officina Batheana, 1798.

30. Bell C: Idea of a New Anatomy of the Brain: Submitted for the Observations of His Friends. London, Strahan and Preston, 1811. (Reprinted by Cranefield PF: The Way in and the Way Out:

François Magendie, Charles Bell and the Roots of the Spinal Nerves. New York, Futura Publishing Co., 1974.)

31. Müller J: Handbuch der Physiologie des Menschen für Vorlesungen. Coblenz, J. Hölscher, 1834, vol 1. (Translated by Baly W, as Elements of Physiology. Philadelphia, Lee and Blanchard, 1843.)

32. Miller EC. Truth, stranger than fiction: Silas Weir Mitchell and phantom limbs. Pharos Alpha Omega Alpha Honor Med Soc. 2011 Autumn;74(4):20-24. PMID: 23256240.

LOU'S CRPS, AMPUTATION, AND MEMORY LOSS STORY
Lou Mortelli

My story will be a tad different than others you have read. It will be written mostly thru the eyes of my husband MJ. I lost my memory in 2008. Without getting into too much detail, I do not remember anything before 2008. So...it will be the abridged or abbreviated version.

To get some of the facts out of the way...I was injured at work in 1988, diagnosed with complex regional pain syndrome (CRPS) had multiple related surgeries before and after my amputation and ultimately a left above-knee amputation (AKA) in 2001. Due to CRPS complications, knee fusing and dark discoloration of the leg, an amputation was performed. Looking back at what I just wrote, it does seem like an oversimplification of a serious time in my life...maybe even a little emotionless. I am not trying to make light of what I went through or what others have gone through in similar situations. Please remember my "memory life" started in 2008, and this goes back to 1988.

When I woke up in October of 2008, I did not know the man who came into the room, the dogs on the bed or even my own name. Then I tried to get up, but something just did not feel right. I looked down...and I only had one leg? Immediately I looked at the man, who was my husband MJ, to see if he had one leg. I know...weird thing to do. Since that day in 2008, I have had to learn so many things. Most people would say "over or again", but for me...it's new and for the first time.

In my situation, I am unable to use a prosthetic and I get around with a manual wheelchair. Even though I have had multiple hand surgeries, I feel I do well in my wheelchair. Although...a day does not go by where someone does not say to me "How come you do not wear a prosthetic?" or "You should get a prostate." No, not a misspelling. Maybe because of 9/11, people feel they can say such things. Other daily issues I face have to do with phantom sensations (feelings of pain, wetness and itchiness) pain and struggling to maintain an upright position in my wheelchair. Pressing down on my stump all day to sit straight is painful mentally and physically.

My life began in 2008, where I had a husband who stood by me...even though he had to struggle with his own memories of our friendship and marriage ruined by my memory loss. I had none of these memories and would have to fall in love with him again. To this day, I find that amazing...why did he stay with me...how does he do it every day? This doesn't even include having an amputee wife in a wheelchair, with CRPS and life-threatening allergies. I am lucky to have MJ in my life.

MY NEW LEFT LEG: LIFE AS AN AMPUTEE WITH CRPS

Eric M. Phillips

I developed complex regional pain syndrome (CRPS) in my left foot and leg on December 7, 1985. I was involved in a car accident. I was a passenger with someone drunk (at the time I did not know he was drunk). I did know that he had a few drinks after work, but I did not know how many. He was the type of person that could drink a lot and still function in life and drive without any problems.

Well, I guess the drinking that he did early that day caught up with him while we were driving to his girlfriend's house that night. He fell asleep behind the wheel. The crazy thing is that I saw the accident coming ahead of time, but there was nothing that I could do. We hit a rock monument on someone's property on the passenger's side of the car, so I took the brunt of the impact. I do remember bracing my left foot into the floorboard of the car at the time of impact, and I felt an electrical jolt go up my left leg and I heard a pop in my lower back. When the EMTs arrived at the scene of the accident, I remember the EMT asking me if I was okay and if I had pain. I think I was in shock from the accident so, I told him I had some pain. He told me to wait until tomorrow morning when I get up, I will be in pain. Boy was this guy right! I was in so much pain. It was a type of pain that I never felt before.

While I was in the ER at the local hospital, they did the routine checks and sent me home. I was informed that the driver of the car had a high blood alcohol level. Too bad that I did not know that before I got into that car that night.

After my accident, I went to see an orthopedic doctor because of the pain in my left foot, leg, and lower back. He was not able to tell me what was wrong with my foot, leg, or lower back, so he just sent me to physical therapy for a few months.

As time went on my foot, leg and lower back were getting worse. After six months the orthopedic doctor told me he could not do anything for me and sent me on my way to fend for myself.

As, we all know most CRPS patients have to see many doctors during the course of their disease. I saw between 20 to 30 doctors in a two-and-half-year span before I was finally diagnosed with CRPS. The sad thing is that the first doctor I saw after my accident, knew I had CRPS but he never informed me.

After my official diagnosis of CRPS, I had many sympathetic nerve blocks (SNB), and Bier blocks, all of which did not provide me with any long-term relief.

As time when on my left foot became deformed. My toes curled under and my ankle turned in. It was difficult to walk, but I did it for three years and one week. At, this time I had my first surgery on December 14, 1988. I had a fusion of my great left toe. After that surgery, my CRPS spread up my leg past my knee. After the spread started, I lost the use of my left leg (for over 20-years).

Over the past 35 years of dealing with my CRPS and back injury, I have had multiple back surgeries that have failed, and ultimately, I had to have an above-knee amputation (AKA) due to infections caused by the CRPS that first developed on February 14, 2007. Dealing with the infections in my foot and leg, I was admitted into the hospital every other month, for a year and a half to help fight these infections with I.V. antibiotics which did not do too much for the infections and they made me feel like crap.

In June of 2008, I was in the hospital again for a week to treat the infections. After being in the hospital for a week, my doctors came into my hospital room to discuss with me that the antibiotics were not working as they hoped they would have to help control the infections. So, they discussed with me my options of what to do next? I was given two options.

- Option one: was to continue with the I.V. antibiotics for another five to six months until the infection killed me.

- Option two: was to have an amputation. Boy, hearing the word AMPUTATION was a big-time wake-up call for me.

I had discussed this new situation with my primary care doctor. I told him that I would have to think about that for a minute. It was a long minute.... Lol! My doctor recommended that I should speak with a vascular surgeon who does amputations. He had referred me to a wonderful and amazing vascular surgeon Doctor MC.

I was fortunate to have met this surgeon. He spent over an hour with me going over my options and discussing the pros and cons of doing this procedure. I had many questions for him regarding my CRPS. I asked the typical questions like do you know what CRPS is? How many patients have you seen with the disease? Have you performed an amputation on CRPS patients before and what were the results? Well, he was honest with me and told me he knew about CRPS, but he never did an amputation on a patient with CRPS. I told him my hopes and fears of doing this surgery. He was open to learning more about CRPS and amputations. This impressed me to know he was willing to learning more about what I was dealing with and he was willing to work with me. He told me that I was in control of the ship when it came to my health and care. After leaving the hospital, I spent the next month beating myself up (mentally) with deciding to do the surgery to amputate my left leg above the knee.

During my month off from the hospital and dealing with my infections, I went to see a Psychologist (which I would highly recommend to anyone thinking of having an amputation). I was fortunate to have met a wonderful Psychologist Doctor B (as I call her) a few years before my surgery. I am so grateful that she helped me in dealing with the fact of having an amputation. She had put it in the best perspective to me. She had asked me if my foot and leg were my friend or enemy now at this time in my life? My answer to her was, it was my enemy; after that conversation, I made my decision to do the surgery. Thank you, Doctor B!

My Amputation

On August 25th and 27th, 2008 I went through the most difficult surgery that I have ever been through in my life. I had to have a two-stage amputation.

One week, before my surgery, I met with my vascular surgeon to discuss what we were going to do for the surgery. At, this point and time the infections were at their worst. I was only sleeping between one to two hours a night due to the pain of the CRPS and the infections. Once, my surgeon saw how bad the infections got, he said that he had to rethink what route he was going to take for my surgery. He said since the infections got worse, he recommended doing a two-stage amputation. As he had explained to me that on the first day, he would amputate my foot at the ankle to let the rest of the infection drain out of my leg for a day. He then asked me if I wanted to stay awake for this first surgery which would be a guillotine cut of the foot at the ankle. He said it would only take 10-minutes to do the procedure. I asked him if he was smoking crack in his pipe? Lol! I told him a big NO! I wanted to be knocked the hell out for the surgery.

Well, I must say that the first part of my amputation surgery went well. To be honest, I felt great not having that infected and painful (for over 20 plus years) foot on my body anymore. I was like a different person laughing and telling jokes to the nurses and doctors. So, on the third day of being in the hospital, I had the second stage of the amputation done. The surgery went well, but I felt more pain than, I had after the first surgery. I knew that it was not going to be an easy ride without having some type of pain.

I was in the hospital for six days. I remember the first time I tried to get out of bed without having my leg. It felt strange, but I was used to not using my left leg to walk for the past 20 plus years, so it was no big deal getting used to being an amputee. I was released from the hospital and went home to finally get some well-deserved rest. As one knows, no one sleeps, while they are in the hospital. I was also looking forward to getting some good home-cooked food from my mom. You know how hospital food can be.

Well, my first night home sleeping in my bed did not go as well as I planned. The moment I got into my bed, I started to get really bad muscle spasms in my stump (which was nicknamed Stumpy by my dear friend Tracey P.).

These spasms lasted six to seven hours. I could not move an inch in my bed without having severe pain in my stump from the spasms. I had called my surgeon's office and I spoke with a doctor who was covering for him over the weekend. I told him what was going on and asked him to phone in a prescription for a muscle relaxant. He said that I would have to drive back to the hospital in Boston to be checked out. I said to him are you crazy? I knew what is going on, and I needed something for the spasms. So, I hung up the phone since I was not getting anywhere with this idiot doctor. I asked my mom to call 911 to take me to the local ER. They came right away and took me to the local hospital. After being there for six hours, they sent me home with a prescription for a muscle relaxant. It did help with the spasms briefly, so I was able to get some sleep.

The next night, the same thing happened to me again. The spasms started back up again. After a few hours of dealing with this again, I had asked my wonderful mother to call 911 again to take me back to the MGH in Boston again to see my surgeon, to figure out what was causing these spasms. Well, the reason for all these spasms was because I had another infection that I had developed above my incision. After finding this out, I was back on I.V. antibiotics for another six days. Thank God that the antibiotics helped with the infection this time. It was well worth staying in the hospital again for another six days.

Finally, I was home and resting in my bed again. Then the fun started with adjusting to my new life of being an amputee with CRPS. For weeks my days were filled with visiting nurses coming in to change the dressings on my stump (stumpy) and checking for any new infections. Thank God I never had another bad infection again. Knock on wood! After a few weeks of being home, I started in-home physical therapy (PT). It was fun learning new ways to do things as an amputee. I was ahead of the game because I live the past 23 years of not using my left leg due to pain, so I was used to using crutches and a wheelchair.

After about a month of in-home PT, I started out-patient PT, at a local place not too far from my home. This is where I started to build up my strength again to get ready to be fitted for my first prosthetic leg.

In, October of 2008, I started the process of being fitted for my first prosthetic socket and microprocessor knee (C-Leg) I gave my new leg a nickname. I call him Lefty. I did not realize how much work goes into making a prosthetic socket. You have to go through a casting process to have a mold of your stump so, they can start creating your socket. It is a very amazing process to witness. I was very fortunate to be referred to Nextstep Bionics and Prosthetics in Warwick RI (I won't name names; you know who you are Lol!). I cannot thank all of the great people at Nextstep for giving me my life back with my new leg.

On November 12, 2008, I got my new left leg and I took my first steps walking after 20 plus years of only walking on one leg. It was a scary feeling taking my first steps on my new prosthetic leg. I felt like Forest Gump! Run Forest Run!!! I had no clue what I was doing, but I did it. I think it was my Dad watching over me that day from heaven. I just wish he was there to see me walking in person. I remember the look on my mom's face when she saw me take my first steps. It was the best thing to view! I saw how happy she was. It made me feel great to see her so happy.

The Battles of Living as an Amputee with CRPS

I have to be honest with everyone reading my story. Having an amputation when you suffer from CRPS is not the first option any patient should think of having done. Yes, I know we all want to get rid of our painful burning or ice-cold limb. If amputation was the first and best option, I think we would all be amputees.

There are many other treatment options that patients can try way before the option of amputation comes into the picture. Usually, amputations are done when the patient reaches the end-stage of the disease (as in my case due to infections). When I was making my decision to have my left leg amputated, I spoke with the late Doctor Hooshmand (my mentor and best friend). I had told him what was going on with my infections. He told me that in his 40-plus years of being a Neurologist, he had only given his blessings on six amputations for CRPS patients. I was the seventh patient he gave the blessing to have the surgery, but it was not without a lot of discussion of the pros and cons of having an amputation when you have CRPS. Doctor Hooshmand has always advocated against this type of surgery in cases of CRPS because he has seen what the long-term effects of CRPS can cause a patient to go through.

As I discussed the pros and cons of doing this amputation with Doctor Hooshmand, I understood the cons of the potential spread of my CRPS, more infections, phantom pain, and the ability to not be able to wear a prosthesis. These are all factors that scared me to death. The pros of having the amputation were that I might be able to use the prosthesis and walk again after 20 plus years. The other pros of having the amputation were to have a better quality of life. This was Doctor Hooshmand's biggest thing he wanted for all his patients, was to have a better quality of life. I know to this day that Doctor Hooshmand gave me his blessings and agreed that doing this surgery was the best thing to do so, I could have a better quality of life. I cannot thank him enough for all his great advice and support over the years and during the time I was having my amputation.

As I tell people it's not easy being an amputee. It can be very painful at times and it can be very challenging and frustrating at times too. It's a lot of work walking on a prosthetic leg for many people including myself.

Most people do not understand what it is like being an amputee. They think that it's great that you had your leg amputated and you have a new prosthetic leg, so now you can walk again. I wish it was that easy. Lol! Little do they know, that we are constantly going through changes with the anatomy of our stumps. I was told in the first year of being an amputee that I may go through at least three to six different sockets. Well, I was lucky I only went through three sockets in my first year. In total over the last 12 years, I have had ten sockets and four knees. I received my fourth new knee (a C-Leg 4) on May 28, 2019, and my tenth socket on March 5, 2020.

Many CRPS patients that have undergone an amputation spend months to years (like myself) going to physical therapy to build up strength in their stumps and whole body. In my case of not walking for over 20 plus years, I had to start all over to learn how to walk on two feet again. I spent two years in physical therapy to get stronger and learn how to use my prosthesis the proper way. I was very fortunate that one of my physical therapists was also an amputee. He was an above-knee amputee just like me. So, who better to learn from than another amputee? I was grateful to spend my time in physical therapy learning how to walk again. I know that I am still learning every day to be the best walker I can after 12 years. I know I will never run again, but I am just happy and grateful I can walk again. 😊

A helpful tip for other newly amputees, the best exercise and way to help with your walking is to go to a supermarket and walk around the store pushing the shopping cart. I find that I do my best walking while pushing the cart. So, I love going food shopping with my wife, because I get some good exercise and it helps improve my walking skills. One thing you have to be careful of is the wheels of the shopping cart. Many times, my prosthetic foot and wheel have had a lot of run-ins over the years. You have to keep an eye out for the wheel of the cart and an eye on your prosthetic foot. It's not a fun feeling when you almost trip because of the wheel hits your foot you cannot feel.

The fun part of having a prosthetic is having my sockets made. After they create the socket, they can take any t-shirt with a design on it and laminate it to the socket. It's a cool process to watch. I have had many cool designs on my sockets over the years. Most people who know me, know that I am a big Todd Rundgren Fan. He is my favorite music artist. I have been following his music since my older brother Michael turned me on to Todd's music in the 1970s. I have had many of Todd's concert t-shirt images on my sockets over the years. Todd has been so kind as to autograph a few of my sockets for me when I have met him at his concerts.

My Pros and Cons of Having an Amputation

The pros of having an amputation for me are being able to wear my prosthesis and having the feeling of being whole again. Every time I put my prosthesis on, I feel like it is part of my body and I can put one foot in front of the other. It's a great feeling! I am very fortunate that I can wear a prosthesis. I know many CRPS patients that have had an amputation and cannot wear a prosthesis for many reasons.

The other pro of having my amputations was that I got rid of my painful useless foot and leg. As I always said my leg just went for the ride with me. Lol! Being an amputee has given me a better quality of life all around with spending time with my wife and our family. Do not get me wrong I have had my share of bad days with my prosthesis. I have had times when my socket has become too loose for me and my leg starts to fall off on me while I am walking or even when I am sitting. These are the things that can happen when you are an amputee. The funniest thing that happened to me one time while I was in physical therapy, my therapist had me try to ride a stationary bike. Well, I got on the bike for the first time in over 20 years, and the next thing I knew my leg fell off. I lost suction in my socket. It was too funny! I was laughing my butt off. But these are some of the things that can happen when you are an amputee. You just have to learn to deal with it and you have to make light of it too. It is part of the learning process. All around in my case, it had been a positive thing for me to have had the amputation done. I have been asked by my relatives and friends if I think I should have done it earlier in my life after my accident and when things got worse? My answer to them was no. I always had the attitude that I would keep my leg as long as I could or until it started to affect my health. Also, I was not ready for it mentally. The month that I took off to make my decision about having the amputation helped me a great deal. I finally came to peace with the idea of having the surgery done the week before my surgery date. The night before the surgery I was totally at peace with myself. I have only questioned my decision once in the past 12 years. It was on my first night home after my surgery when I had those awful spams in my stump for six to seven hours straight. This was the only time I said to myself why did I do this? Since then, I have never looked back at the past. I now only look towards the future. I am fortunate that I live in this day and age. Just think if this was a hundred years ago or more, I would be walking on a wooden leg made by Peg Leg himself. Lol! I am lucky to have such a wonderful prosthetic microprocessor knee and carbon-fiber socket with a cool design on it.

The cons of having my amputation. My number one con since my amputation is that I developed phantom pain (or as I call it "The Phantom"). The other cons are worrying about getting infections again, and the small things like having issues with my prosthesis not fitting properly and having to get a new socket made, and getting uses to it all over again. This issue can be a pain at times, but it can be fixed, unlike having phantom pain. So, in my case, I feel like the pros outweigh the cons.

Phantom Pain

In my opinion, phantom pain is the most brutal type of pain one can endure. I feel that phantom pain is worse than CRPS pain. I have had phantom pain from day one after my surgery. Some amputees are lucky that they may have phantom pain for a short time after their surgery or never at all. In my case, I have it regularly. Phantom pain is strange at times. It can come and goes anytime it likes and it never gives you a warning. Sometimes a few days before a storm is coming in, the "Phantom" shows up, it can happen at any time during the day or night. It can happen while you are having dinner or in the middle of the night when you are sleeping. It can last for a few hours to a few days. My longest battle with "The Phantom" was for 36 hours straight with no sleep. Talk about being a zombie! The strange thing about phantom pain, is it changes locations on my foot and leg every time. Sometimes it will attack three toes, then there are times I feel it just in my great toe, and then there are times I feel it on the bottom of my foot or in parts of my leg. The wired thing is that in 12 years I have only felt it in my knee six-times. The other things I have felt when I have had phantom pain are the areas where I had my infections, the screw that was in my great toe, and where they did the first amputation at my ankle.

Over the years there has been much debate between what we call phantom pain and phantom sensations. In my opinion, they are both the same. When I get the so-called phantom sensations, they are still painful. So why classify it just as a sensation? To me pain is pain. Phantom pain or phantom sensations are all the same. Painful! Some people and doctors think that phantom pain is all in your head. Well, like all pain sensations you do feel them in your head. When they amputate your limb, they do not remove the nerves that were attached to that limb. The nerves are still there connected to your brain. They place the rest of the nerves into your residual limb; hence they are still connected to your body and brain. That is why you still feel the pain. Like I say to people, nerves are not like a wiring harness in a car that can be removed and replaced. When they amputate a limb, they do not remove the nerve that was connected from the brain to the amputated limb.

When I get phantom pain, it feels like I am being repeatedly stabbed over and over, all day and night long. Nothing helps with this type of pain. I have tried different pain medications which do not help the pain at all. So, I listen to my favorite music artist (Todd Rundgren) to try to keep my mind off the pain. I use Todd's music as my form of bio-feedback to help cope with my phantom pain. I am grateful to Todd and his great music.

People ask me how do I cope and deal with phantom pain? My answer is I just ride the wave out. There is nothing that I can do about it or for it. I cannot control when I get it. As I say it has a mind of its own. It comes and goes as it pleases.

Conclusion

I want everyone to know that I do not advocate amputation for CRPS treatment. It is not a form of treatment. Amputation should only be considered when a patient is at the end-stage of the disease and every other form of treatment has been tried. Twelve-years ago, when I was in my 23rd-year of having CRPS, I had reached that end-stage of the disease, due to un-controllable infections. At that time, I had no choice to have the surgery. It was either life or limb, and I picked life over limb. I figured hey, I can get a new cool-looking bionic leg out of the deal. Why not! Lol!

I do not regret having my amputation. I am very grateful to my wife, my Mom and (Dad watching over me from Heaven), my family, friends, doctors, therapists, and my wonderful prosthetists that have helped me over the past 12 years.

Being able to walk again has been a huge blessing and it has made me feel like a new person again. It has made a big impact on my life for the best. It has improved my quality of life, just like Doctor Hooshmand wanted for me. I have been lucky and blessed in my life. A little over two years ago I married the love of my life. My wonderful and beautiful wife Mercedes. She is my rock and she is the one who is always there to get me out walking and doing things in life. I cannot thank her enough for all her love and support. Thank you, my sweet love!

So, my advice to any CRPS patient who thinks that having an amputation is the answer, please think long and hard before you make that decision. It's a big decision to make and it's a permanent one too. Do your research. Talk to others who have been through it. I was very fortunate that I have a very close and great friend of mine who has CRPS and is an amputee too. She was a great resource and friend to me when I was going through making my decision to have my surgery. I cannot thank her enough. 😊

Having CRPS and being an amputee is just a part of my life now. Having the amputation saved my life and it has given me a better quality of life too. We need to have more research on CRPS and more research on the effects of amputation in CRPS patients. We need to educate the medical community and spread more awareness on CRPS. This has been my mission for the past 32 years. I feel that we are all part of this big RSD-CRPS Puzzle. We all need to work together to help find the answers and maybe someday find a cure for CRPS, so no one will ever have to suffer from this painful disease ever again. Please stay well and keep positive! 😊 Eric

20-SECONDS LATER
Anita Carden

It was the 17th of September 2015. I had awoken that day in one of the most beautiful places on earth, Mount Cook, New Zealand. As my husband and I had been touring NZ for three weeks, our holiday was coming to an end and we had saved the best till last. We got out of bed on this beautiful morning and got ready to do a hike to the Tasman Glacier. We checked out of our accommodation and drove the short distance up the valley to the bottom of the glacier. We got out of the car and started up the rocky path to the viewing platform at the top. It was a short walk, in comparison to the other glaciers in NZ and we were looking forward to adding this hike to our list.

The view from the top was exquisite. We looked down onto beautiful Tasman Glacier and it was breathtaking. After standing there and taking it all in, we turned to head back down the rocky path back to the bottom. Luke went ahead of me and started heading down first. Before I ventured down, I stood at the top taking in the incredible view of the hooker valley. The icy air was nipping at my cheeks and I could hear an avalanche on the other side of the mountain. To say it was a perfect moment is an understatement. I just stood there taking it all in. It was serene. In a sense it was unreal. Could it get any better than this?

So, 20 seconds later my life as I knew it had changed forever.

I started back down the rocky path watching every step as I went, the path was uneven and I was careful to make sure I stayed upright. So, 20 seconds into heading back from the glacier, I rolled my left ankle. Not a sprain, just a roll. It was very insignificant and at the time did not hurt at all. It was just a little stumble and I kept walking down the uneven path. When I got back to the car, we drove onto Hanmer Springs where we booked into our accommodation for the night.

The next morning, I awoke to awful pain in my left ankle. On inspection I saw it was black, blue and purple and very swollen, I couldn't bear weight at all. We drove onto Christchurch where we went to the hospital to get a pair of crutches and get my ankle checked out. I was told to keep it wrapped and to stay off it and it will be ok in a few days.

The following day we flew home and the morning after I went to see a GP. He did a Doppler test thinking it may be deep vein thrombosis from flying, and also an X-ray. Both came back clear. When I had no relief in a few days I saw another GP. He took blood tests and did an ultrasound but that also came back clear. The pain was terrible and I knew something was wrong but neither of the doctors I'd seen had any clue what was wrong.

By this point, my GP who had been away when I got home from NZ had returned so I booked an appointment with her. She referred me to a neurologist who did very extensive blood tests but who also had no clue what was wrong. I still could not put my foot to the floor so was still tied to crutches. It was now six months since "that hike".

At this point, the pain had spread to above my knee and I had a purple rash that accompanied the pain. It was in a neat line above my knee, I could see where the pain "ended". It was just so baffling to me. My leg was dead and useless and I had to carry it everywhere. It was at this point that my limb felt like it did not belong to me. It felt alien and I wanted it gone. The mental torture was as bad as the physical pain and I started having panic attacks where I'd rip all my clothes off feeling as though I was suffocating. I was desperate to get the alien limb off and having these times where I'd end up completely naked was embarrassing, to say the least, I am thankful I was in the car with my husband at the time and he would get me home and dressed again.

I was then referred to a vascular surgeon who was shocked to feel the difference in temperature and color. On the outside my leg was purple and cold but, on the inside, it burned like fire. "Move it or lose it," he said. "You do not understand," I said. "I cannot even put my foot to the floor let alone bear weight".

By this time, it was May 2017, and my knee had developed a contracture and stayed perpetually bent. Crutches had become a part of my life and I was often in a wheelchair. The pain raged on and the rash would change color and texture every day. I would wake a night trying to tear my leg off which only added to the pain. At this point, I saw a rheumatologist who said "That is complex regional pain syndrome (CRPS)". I said "What's that?" He explained it as best he could and I was relieved to put a name to it. He showed me photos of other people with it and everything started to fall into place. He immediately got on the phone to a pain clinic and two weeks later I started with the team there. By this time, it was June 2017.

My first appointment with the multi-disciplinary pain clinic confirmed the diagnosis of CRPS. I immediately started a program wherein the four doctors involved with my treatment tried to halt the beast. My team consisted of a head doctor, a nurse, a physiotherapist, and a Psychologist. They started mirror therapy immediately but every time I looked in the mirror at my leg, I would vomit. They gave me an app on my phone that was designed to get me to choose between photos of the left and right feet but when I looked at it, I couldn't tell the left foot from the right and I would be nauseated. The more I looked at the app in trying to identify left from right, I'd get to the point of vomiting. Then they tried to prick my leg and asked me to identify where I felt it but I had no clue where they had touched. Ankle? Knee? Thigh? All I knew is that they touched my leg, but where?? At this point, it was clear my brain had rejected my limb. My leg was now bleeding every day. Air would hurt it, water made it bleed, clothes would stick to it, loud noises hurt, I was a mess. I was given medication after medication but nothing worked, in fact, everything I tried made me really sick.

I spent six months with the pain clinic and although they wanted to do aggressive physical therapy, I couldn't put my foot to the floor and the twice they pushed me to bear weight, I ended up vomiting and passed out on the ground. I told them to take my leg off and they told my husband because no medication was working, it was all in my head and sent me to a psychiatrist. Doctor T.D., was a great psychiatrist and when I told her that medication did not work, she immediately did a DNA test which returned showing that I am allergic to all medications!! At last, I had proof that the meds I'd been given did not in fact work. It wasn't "all in my head".

At this point, my GP who was in agreement with my request for amputation found a pain specialist in Adelaide, Doctor P.C., who had done an amputation for CRPS, so I made an appointment to see him. I saw him in December 2017, the month I left the pain clinic.

At my first appointment, he was shocked at the extent that CRPS had taken hold. Even though he was booked out for six months, he told me to be back in Adelaide on the 17th of January 2018, where he did a sympathectomy and a sciatic nerve block. Both were unsuccessful. As Doctor P.C., was a private specialist and my insurance had not yet kicked in, he referred me to the public sector to a professor of a pain clinic in a major hospital in Sydney to have a trial of a spinal cord stimulator (SCS).

I had my first appointment with professor C.B., in April 2018, and he did an infusion of pamidronate (a bisphosphonate), but this just made me really ill. I was back a month later for a trial of a spinal cord stimulator which was supposed to be an eight-day trial, but when I had no relief the morning after they put it in, he took it out the next day. It was a new SCS that had just become available and he said if it was going to work it would have provided relief immediately.

At this point, I told him I wanted it off and showed him a folder full of information I had printed off on a study done at the University hospital in the Netherlands. Even though the numbers were low in the case study, it showed a high success rate for amputation for CRPS. I found out later that the information I gave him changed his opinion on amputation for this hideous syndrome and paved the way for others coming after me to have an amputation if all other treatments had failed.

As I had formed a connection with Doctor P.C., in Adelaide, I returned to him where he approved an above-knee amputation. So, on the 21st of June 2018, I said good riddance to my evil limb. As I was wheeled into theatre, my surgeon walked across to me and he held my hand as he spoke to me about nothing in particular while my anesthetist got everything ready to put me to sleep. Then the surgeon got a black marker out of his pocket and put a line just above the "rash". I knew from my research that the amputation had to be above the level of allodynia and I knew that the mark he had just drawn on my thigh was going to change my life. As I stared at the lights above my head, I knew I was about to be set free...

The morning after my operation, I threw back the covers, and there in front of me sat my stump that I immediately connected with. At last, I was free and the relief was overwhelming. The limb I was born with that had turned on me was gone and I found myself staring at the place it had been. I put my hands around the bandage and held my stump in my hands while relief washed over me. It was the cutest little thing, this soft little residual limb that just sat there in my hands, I was overwhelmed that now my new life starts with this little guy and the evil limb was gone. My stump belonged to me, my leg did not. Mentally and emotionally, I had been put back together again.

I had a new lease on life. Doctor P.C., kept nerve blocks up to me so I had no pain at all. Getting up and down to the bathroom was now a breeze as was turning over in bed, getting dressed, and moving around on crutches.

About four days after my operation, phantom pain started. It's hard to describe just how excruciating it is. It was constant and severe and it took my sleep. The team at the hospital told me that it was likely it would not last but being in the thick of it, it was difficult to see light at the end of the tunnel.

After 10-days in the hospital, I was discharged as a new woman. I had joined the amputee community and I was free. One would have to live with a CRPS limb to understand what that means. I'd lost a leg but I left the hospital feeling whole.

Two-weeks later we left Adelaide for the long 2,000 km trip home. The trip home was so much easier because the CRPS pain was gone. I could sit in the car for hours on end without pain. Phantom pain continued to be an issue but I worked really hard for two-months and cleared it with EFT (emotional freedom technique) and mirror therapy.

On the 2nd of August, I was cast for my first socket, six weeks after my amputation. Two weeks after that on the 16th I took my first steps on two legs and it was the best feeling in the world! I worked hard in PT and put my heart and soul into regaining my mobility. As my stump changed shape and started shrinking, I was cast again for another socket, then another and another! I just kept shrinking and stabilizing the more I walked in my socket and I made sure every day I'd do a 2 kilometer (km) walk on the beach. It was the best feeling getting back to my beach walks after not being able to get onto the beach for so long.

Now, two and a half years after relinquishing my CRPS limb, my life is so much better. CRPS is a thief. It takes without asking, and it ruins lives. I was determined to take back what it took from me and since my amputation, I have been back to NZ three times, and I live an active life.

It is my hope that doctors will acknowledge that CRPS is more than just a pain syndrome. It gets into your head; it gets under your skin. It affects every part of the body and mind. I hope that doctors will start to listen so they can understand just what a person with CRPS goes through on a daily basis.

I may have lost a limb but I've gained so much more. CRPS tried to beat me, but I won.

"IT NEVER OCCURRED TO ME THAT ONE DAY I WOULD WAKE UP SICK AND NEVER GET BETTER"

L.E.

It never occurred to me when I went to bed on March 6, 2019, that I would wake up to the worst day of my life, a traumatic right-hand pinky amputation followed by Complex Regional Pain Syndrome (CRPS). While we were visiting my fiancé's family in Georgia, my accident happened early in the morning on March 7, 2019, around 6:45 am when I was trying to separate my dogs from each other, as they were in a horrible territorial fight.

I have two decent sized dogs, a Husky and an Akita, I am only 5' tall, and I was trying to pull them apart from each other, my hand slipped off the husky's silky fur while I was grabbing her which caused my hand to fall into the biting zone causing the part from the nail up of my right pinky to be removed and never found. After cleaning the wound as best they could, I started passing out while being rushed to the closest emergency room (ER) by my fiancé and his mother. I was in emergency surgery by 10:30 am, as the doctor had to perform another surgery before mine, I thought this would be the end, but it's only the beginning.

This accident already pushed our plans of going back home to Maine back a few weeks, as I was in occupational therapy towards the end of April 2019, I started noticing a nail growth, and it was very painful. Another doctor performed a nail removal procedure on May 24, 2019, and we traveled back home to Maine at the beginning of June 2019. I saw my primary care provider who referred me to an orthopedist, before I even saw the orthopedist, another nail grew in not even giving my dissolvable stitches time to dissolve. The doctor who performed the nail removal procedure in May said it was not guaranteed that another nail would not grow back, but I did not think it would grow in so quickly.

It was the weekend before I went to see the orthopedist, and I had to soak the stitches/nail in water and trim it myself because it was getting caught on everything, which was very painful. When I saw the orthopedist on June 26, 2019, he was quite confused why they did not take more off my pinky, so there would be no nail growth, so we arranged for corrective amputation surgery on July 12, 2019.

Twelve days after my surgery, he pulled the "Frankenstein stitches" from my poor pinky (as if it had not gone through enough), I screamed bloody murder the whole time, and he was confused why it hurt, and I was bleeding a lot, making it difficult for him to see, so he kept having to wipe it he then numbed it when he was done. I was trying to ask him about medications as I discussed with him before this surgery. My whole hand was always in pain and not just my pinky. He told me to google complex regional pain syndrome (CRPS) and to go across the street to the drugstore to get some Lidocaine and that was the end of that appointment.

I left that appointment first of all in more pain than I came in with and second of all so confused/angry with how that appointment just went. I called my primary care's office and told them what happened and that I want a new doctor immediately.

I saw a new orthopedist in August 2019 and thank god I did; she started me on Gabapentin and gave me a referral for an Electromyography (EMG), and a referral for a finger prosthetic. By, September 2019 the pain in my entire hand also traveled to my wrist, and by October, the pain continued to spread to my elbow. I had my appointment with a neurologist for an

EMG towards the end of October where he diagnosed me with CRPS. The orthopedist received the neurologist's notes and referred me to physical therapy and the pain management department in her office.

In November, when I started physical therapy, the pain had continued to spread to my Deltoid, and I also saw the first pain specialist at the beginning of November. She prescribed an antidepressant (Elavil) which I had a horrible time taking it. It felt like I was in a Tim Burton movie the whole time I was on it, and she wanted to prescribe others which I was not a fan of as it's not solving my pain.

By December the pain had spread to my shoulder blade, and I saw the first pain specialist again at the beginning of December who referred me to the second pain specialist which I had an appointment at the end of December.

In December, I finally got my finger prosthetic (PIP Driver from Naked Prosthetics) and it was a lifesaver for protecting my pinky, and allowing me to try to use my hand more natural. At first, it was awkward, but I got used to it by the end of the weekend, although it is not a real finger and it does slide off easy with water; it helps my pain a lot more than in the hours I do not wear it.

By January 2020, the pain had continued to spread from my shoulder blade with the line of pain to the right of my spinal cord. I did not even know what kind of doctor I needed to see anymore? So, since a plastic surgeon originally did my first surgery in March 2019, and I had my primary care doctor send a referral to a new plastic surgeon.

I live on the Canadian Border in Maine, so there are not too many specialists up here, especially the ones I need to see, so I had to drive the entire state of Maine (six hours) to Portland to see this plastic surgeon. I thought I would get answers only to be disappointed. I had a 4:00 pm appointment and when I was finally called back; it was almost 5:00 pm, and the doctor came in the room with his jacket on like he's already warming up his car and told me, there is nothing we can do for the pain, and that it should not spread anymore, and I should stop smoking and stop my caffeine intake.

By February the pain spread from the right of my spine up to my neck and since I was in physical therapy, my therapist suggested that I try dry needling and that another one of their locations offer this, so I tried this in February 2020, only to find out the dry needling "aggravated the beehive".

I also saw the second pain specialist again in February, and he increased my Gabapentin intake from 1,500 mg to 2,100 mg and suggested we try a stellate ganglion block injection. I was supposed to have this done in March 2020, but because of COVID-19 all hospital and doctors' visits were limited to certain things and an injection was not one of them.

Since I was in so much pain, my primary care doctor also prescribed me a muscle relaxer and suggested I try Osteopathic Manipulative Treatment (OMT). Also, because of the pandemic, OMT treatment was not the type of appointment doctors were taking at the time. I was going insane with not knowing where to turn to next, and how to deal with my pain, and how to deal with my decline of independence.

So, my primary care doctor also referred me to behavioral health. I finally found another doctor that could perform Osteopathic Manipulative Treatment (OMT) during this time, but I would have to switch primary care to him instead, so I had nothing to lose at this point, so I switched. I was so excited when I finally got a call from my pain specialist in May saying they can start scheduling injection appointments again, so I made an appointment for May 20, 2020, and on the same day, since I have to travel three hours round trip to see these doctors, I also had my first new primary care appointment.

I had the injection done after my new primary care appointment and when I got home that evening; I was eating dinner when suddenly both sides under my chin started going numb, and it spread to both sides of my jaws into my bottom lip then to my top lip, then I couldn't swallow and then the numbness was creeping up into my cheekbones. I called the doctor in a panic and told him what was going on (I felt like I was having a heart attack, and I was only 25 at the time), since this was not a normal side effect. He wanted me to go get checked out at the ER, and the CT scan came back normal. I went home, but could not sleep all night because of so much pain in my neck and having persisting numbness in my face. Ever since this happened, the right side of my neck is so tense it is also affecting my Trapezius muscle, causing me so much pain even laying down.

I saw the pain specialist a week after the injection which he referred me to physical therapy, and he wanted me to decrease my Gabapentin but did not tell me how to do it. Eventually, I was only placed on Cymbalta. I decreased one pill every day out of the 2,100 mg Gabapentin and a week later when I literally could not get out of bed because I was in so much pain. I started the Cymbalta, and it also gave me adverse reactions, so after a week of that I was done with it. I got back on Gabapentin two days after being off of it because I could not handle the pain, yet I did not want to be on the 2,100 mg I was previously on because I felt like a zombie 24/7, and it did not help my pain, so I dosed myself with 900-1,200 mg of Gabapentin.

I have been seen by my new primary care and I had Osteopathic Manipulative Treatment for three treatments and trigger point injections, and I am still in so much pain. He has since referred me to another doctor (physical medicine and rehabilitation) in Scarborough, ME, which is also

61

pretty much six hours away from me. I took this trip to see this doctor in September 2020 since then I have switched to Lyrica 225 mg which he now wants me to increase to 350 mg since the pain is still very persistent, he also referred me again to physical therapy for a "new muscle memory plan" that he is working on with my physical therapist.

It's almost the end of 2020, and I have been in persistent pain since March 2019, and it's pretty miserable, but I try to not let it affect me daily. The behavioral health appointments that I have been going to since the end of April 2020, are helping me deal with things. Even though having CRPS and being an amputee has dramatically changed my life, I realized it gave me such strength I never knew I had before. I did not finish college and because of the strength all of this has given me; I decided to take a paralegal certificate course to better myself, and I have surprised myself with how well I have done with the tight deadlines and ample reading. Although it's tough, I feel like I am not "myself" anymore, I have slowly lost my independence by the month and there was nothing I could do about it. I have "failed" out of physical therapy for the past year.

My pain has caused me to work part-time instead of full time, my hours only decreasing by the months to barely 16 hours a week. I have had to change the way I do a lot of things, for example, my typing style, so instead of "normal" typing, I have to "two-finger peck" on the keyboard. They label CRPS as the "suicide disease", but even though CRPS takes so much out of me and every day and night is a challenge, I try to always think "it could be worse" and in fact, it could. There are people out there with CRPS who have taken their lives, I do not know any, but reading their stories is heartbreaking and my heart feels for them and especially the family they left behind. I do not know where to go from here and I know my CRPS and

62

amputation have decreased my quality of life, but I refuse to be on painkillers because I know my pain is BEYOND that point.

I am trying a chronic pain workbook with my therapist, and it has helped tremendously, but when I'm stressed out or a lot is thrown at me at once it is very hard to incorporate the new coping mechanisms, so I am going to try Lexapro to hopefully be able to manage myself since I feel like I am just losing control at this point. My pain has been so persistent for so long in so many ways I cannot even believe I lived through all this nonsense; it almost feels like a dream or nightmare that never seems to end. I live in a medical marijuana state and when I got my medical card, the doctor suggested I try micro-dosing twice a day with a CBD and THC 50/50 tincture, I have found micro-dosing twice a day with this tincture helped alleviate the "tightness" of the pain. Since I have had all these changes in medicines, I have stopped micro-dosing, so I can see if the medicines are doing their jobs. I also ingest or smoke marijuana to help the pain, I have found this to be the most helpful solution for my pain "tightness" and mental state in comparison to all the medications these doctors want me to "try", I am sick of the "medicine head" these prescriptions give me! I simply want my pain to be gone, but I know that's not going to happen as quickly as I would like it to, but at least some actual pain relief would be AMAZING! It's now February 2021, and I had to get neck x-rays done (remember this all started with a traumatic finger amputation) since my doctors are scratching their heads with how to move forward with a plan that will work this time. I hope they do not see something because who wants something to be wrong right, but at the same time I do hope they see something because I am in a tremendous amount of pain from my finger and hand creeping up my arm into my shoulder, neck, and back. It just does not make sense to me anymore. Why is CRPS so complicated? I guess that's why they call it COMPLEX Regional Pain Syndrome, right?

WALKING THROUGH FIRE

Lauren Malinowitzer

It was the year 2000, and I was in my last year of high school, and I was about to turn 18-years-old. One summer afternoon after playing a friendly game of kickball, I heard a cracking sound in my right ankle. Suddenly, every step I took there was this terrible cracking. In hindsight, I wish I had left the cracking. I was taken to a foot doctor who says, based on films you have osteochondritis dissecans, and we need to do an arthroscopy.

The surgery was scheduled and performed. After the surgery was completed, I was suffering from terrible pain. One night I decided to go to the emergency room. After imaging, they let me know that a piece of the tool used during surgery remained inside my joint. The orthopedic surgeon was called and the surgery was scheduled to remove this foreign object.

During the removal procedure, tendons and ligaments were torn in the process. From this day forward, my life had taken a very unexpected turn. I would now be in constant pain. I had over 30 procedures just to keep me on my feet.

After my first surgery in 2001, I developed symptoms of complex regional pain syndrome (CRPS). Unfortunately, I did not officially receive a diagnosis of CRPS until 2007.

In 2018, things took another terrible turn. I began to have necrosis in my right talus. The doctor I was seeing told me he thought a 3D-talus replacement was the best thing for me. That it would give me back my range of motion and mobility. I had a CT Scan and then the surgery to have the 3D- talus implanted.

From the moment I woke up I knew my life as I knew it was over. I now had pain that was beyond measure. I was no longer able to walk or weight bear. My foot was now a mixture of blue and red. I was told to rest and let it heal. So, 28 weeks later I was still not walking. A new Image was taken showing the implant has shifted.

Another procedure was done to tighten ligaments around the implant. Ten more weeks of healing, and I was still unable to walk.

At, this time I was sent to see another specialist, who informed me that there was no saving my foot. The pulse in the foot has become very weak. The CRPS has taken over the entire foot and ankle, which made it unable for me to move at all. Every touch was excruciating.

After sitting in a recliner for a year, I am now in the deepest depression of my life. I am now contemplating taking my own life. I was living off of hydrocodone 10/325 around the clock. Furthermore, I was sleeping 21 hours a day. I no longer could work, and I was placed on disability. I could no longer live like this.

Finally, I was sent to the Hospital of Special Surgery. The Doctor explained to me that in order to have my life back this foot needed to be removed.

My amputation was scheduled for September 9, 2019. I would have what is called an osseointegration amputation (this involves implanting a metal anchor directly to the bone of an amputated limb that extends out of the residual limb).

As soon as the procedure was over, I no longer had the pain, and I was no longer hostage to a useless limb. This surgery has given my mobility, and my life back. I am now a right below-the-knee amputee (BK).

Over the last 20 years, I have participated in many procedures:

I have had 12-rounds of ketamine infusions, a Medtronic lumbar SCS with 16 panels, Medtronic cervical SCS, Abbott SCS, Abbott DRG, Sympathetic Nerve Blocks, and Radiofrequency ablation (RFA).

I am the founder and president of CRPS-AMPUTEE WARRIORS 501c3. I do everything in my power to let people know that amputation is another cure.

Please visit my support pages on Facebook:

Facebook page:

www.facbook.com/pg/crpsamputeewarriors/community/

Non-Profit- CRPS Amputee Warrior 501c3

Personal page:

www.facebook.com/crpsamputeewarrior/

HOW A FRACTION OF A SECOND CHANGED MY LIFE

Chris Whitman

My journey with complex regional pain syndrome (CRPS) started on the morning of September 10, 2013, when I was working as a clinch press operator. For those that are unfamiliar with a clinch press operator, I made steel parts for airbags. I had been having problems for two weeks before that morning, with one of the sensors on the machine not picking up one of the bolts to press into the steel part. It kept shutting down my machine as the bolt was getting stuck millimeters away from the sensor picking it up. I told my boss it was still doing it and the time was 8:15am. He told me to go get the head quality control engineer, to see if it was the part or the machine causing the problem?

I went over to ask B the head quality control engineer to look at my machine. When B and I got to my machine he asked me to run it so he could see in person what the issue was. Sure, enough first part stopped. There were three safety gates on the machine and a manual shut-off. He asked me to shut the machine down and get him the part so that he could check the measurements on it. When any safety gate is open at all, the whole machine would shut down. I opened the safety gate where the part was and as I opened the safety gate it should have shut the machine down. That's not what happened, instead at 8:29 a.m., as I grabbed the part the bolt dropped into place and the sensor picked it up, for whatever reason. As it picked up the bolt it caused the press to come down in an attempt to press the bolts to the part. B freaked out, one he could not figure out the machine moved and two if I was okay.

As soon as it happened, I instantly said ouch and yanked my hand out of the press. Since it was nothing more than an ouch, I walked back to the QC

67

room with him, but my hand started hurting so I stuck it in my pocket. B was asking me if I was okay and I said yes. The pain started getting worse, and I said I'm going to the restroom.

On my way to the restroom, I felt something wet on that hand, thinking maybe it was sweat I pulled it out and it was blood. Where the press and the part smashed my hand between both it cut straight through the index finger and middle finger. I ran to the sink and instantly started running water over it as it did not look bad, just a lot of blood. As I'm running water over my fingers I notice I could see my bone on my index finger, and I had no movement in it. I stood there for 15 minutes trying to get the bleeding to stop.

Finally, the third-shift supervisor came in and saw it, and ran to get the safety team. They wrapped it up and got the bleeding to stop almost. I was taken to their urgent care to have a tetanus shot and have it examined. They also did the routine drug and alcohol test because it was a work accident.

As the doctor cleaned it out, I had no movement, but tons of pain. He said it had cut my tendons in my index finger and I probably broke bones in multiple fingers. I was told I needed to go to the emergency room right away. The safety guy drove me back to work instead, as he did not know what to do. So, I drove myself to the hospital and was fired for that.

The hospital said there was no tendon tear or broken bones and I was to follow up with the hand surgeon in the morning. I went to see Doctor Al who was an orthopedic specialist. He said to me you have torn your tendons and your index finger was nearly completely cut off but stopped halfway through the bone. How this was not seen at the hospital, I will never know?

So, I was rushed the next day into surgery to fix the tendons in the index finger that I still had no movement in it, yet the pain was just getting stronger by the second.

The surgery was a success and the doctor said I would regain movement and the pain would subside. Well, it did not! After two months of seeing him, the tip of my index finger started to turn inward, toward my palm and the pain was nothing I had ever felt before. The burning felt like pure fire knives cutting through my hand, arm, and neck was so debilitating, and he could not figure out the pain or the movement.

I had a follow up a week later where he had consulted his colleagues. He said to me, Mr. Whitman you have reflex sympathetic dystrophy (RSD) or what is now called complex regional pain syndrome (CRPS). As my wife and I sat there dumbfounded, as we had never heard of it. He starts to explain that when the machine cut through the index finger it damaged my nerve causing it to miss-fire and stay stuck on sending and receiving pain signals.

I was then told there was no cure or true treatment, and that he was sorry that I was his first case of CRPS. Then comes the bureaucracy of workers comp as CRPS is the highest claim next to death in the state of Ohio and were going to fight the hell out of it.

So, for the next two years, I was sent to a ton of workers comp doctors and specialists to discredit the diagnosis, as well as seeing my doctor's all saying no, this is exactly what it is.

I went through bone scans, temperature checks, mobility, basically tortured. This went on for over two years. My index finger by this time had curled to the palm with no use and my other fingers followed. I eventually lost all use of my arm too.

I was denied any treatment for those years as I had to prove to them that I was not lying as their doctors were saying I was. The day finally came to go to court to get everything added to my claim, so I could start getting treatment. I won everything, but it was bittersweet, as in those two-years I lost everything. I lost the use of the hand and my arm was useless. I also lost my house and became homeless, and I ruined the relationship between my kids and me because of the pure agony I was in. Right before I was evicted due to worker's compensation was not paying for anything until all court matters were finished.

I was hallucinating, hearing things, trying to amputate my finger and hand with a knife. I treated my wife horribly and did not want to be that person to the people I love. I had lost all hope of ever getting any help. One morning I took every pill I had in the house while my wife was out. I was done and I could not do it anymore. I committed suicide and my wife found me. She said it took them thirty-minutes just to get me back.

I was in ICU for a couple of weeks and woke up so mad at her and I resented her for not letting me die. It was selfish of me! Not realizing she had to watch them bring her husband back to life for thirty-minutes and still not knowing if I would live or have brain damage.

I slept in my car for an entire winter and it just happened to be the coldest ever on record. I had no heat in my car. Not that it mattered as I did not have gas to run the car either. Cold weather is the worst enemy for a CRPS patient. I had my wife stay with her friend as she did not need to suffer with me.

I finally got a place again that spring and was able to go see an orthopedic doctor who sent me to a specialist to get treatments as he helped document the changes of muscle atrophy, and color and temp changes.

He gave me Percocet that did help with a lot of the joint pain and Lyrica for the CRPS pain. I also had mental health added to my claim for PTSD, depression, and anxiety from it all. I had every injection under the sun done to me by the pain specialist he sent me to, who loved to torture me as I told her they just made it worse.

She started putting me under for them to do the blocks, and one time she had the bright idea to try and straighten the finger, I woke straight up out of it, screaming in immense pain and she had re-broken the finger and ripped all the scars open.

Finally, she believed me. I started researching for myself as I was being offered the spinal cord stimulator (SCS) as my cure-all and holy savior. I did the test stimulator and had minor success. I found Doctor S.H., at the Cleveland Clinic, who was the head of the pain management. He was world-renowned in his CRPS research and treatment. I thought it was my miracle at three-years in.

I went back to see him and he mentioned to me all the blocks and injections I had (with bad results) and he mentioned to me about the trial stimulator I had which only provided me with some ease of my pain. He referred me to see the head neurologist at the Cleveland Clinic to put the permanent stimulator in my neck which required the cutting of eight vertebrae in half and drilling sixteen leads and screws into the neck and run the leads down the arm. It was the worst surgery I ever had and I have had a lot in my life. I had a four-hour ride home and could not even move. I was on the couch for two-months before I healed and they could turn it on and started to program it. When they programmed it, I started getting electrocuted anytime I moved. The representative from St. Jude did not care and just shut it off. The paddle connected to my neck had broken off inside my neck and all sixteen leads became one big knot around my spine. I walked around for three-years before I found a doctor that would remove it as the neurologist that implanted it had left the Cleveland Clinic and Ohio. I still to this day wake up every morning with what feels like a spinal fluid headache and I cannot get it checked out as it's not part of my claim.

So, Doctor S.H., sent me to the top hand surgeon to see if he could help my hand? The time to do anything had passed. My option was either amputating the whole hand or just the index finger and hope with it removed I could start to get the other fingers to work again.

Yes, I begged him to take it. He could not because of worker's comp having to approve everything and it took forever. I could not take it and started sawing the finger off on the four-hour ride home. With the pain I had, I could not do it anymore and not even be able to use my hand or arm.

My wife convinced me to stop. Finally, in February of 2017, I had the index finger and metacarpal to the wrist removed and I was sent for physical therapy yet again. It was too painful to even touch the hand or arm. Doctor SH, retired from Cleveland Clinic and I was sent back to Doctor P, my physician of record to treat me more. I had one option left which was the pain pump.

I went for the trial and I woke up with true tears of joy for the first time in years because I truly felt a little bit of pain relief for first time in many years. I said I want the pump! They set up the operation, and were able to get it all approved. By the time I got home, it had busted loose under my skin. It's barely turned on at this point as it had to heal, to program it to a therapeutic level. I went back into surgery to have it replaced. Two days later the same thing happened again, it became detached under the skin and the pump was trying to come through the scar and skin. This

72

happened five times. Finally, they had to remove it as my body just kept rejecting it. I was defeated! I did not want to live anymore! The Percocet helped a lot but not enough.

So, I played Xbox a lot before my injury and wanted my hand back. If I could not live without pain, I at least wanted to use it. I started trying to play my X-box again and started at three seconds of holding and using the controller and I started seeing improvement as much as the pain killed me to do it. I moved up from three seconds to ten, to a minute and so forth! No matter the pain I pushed through and got 40 percent muscle mass back in my arm and hand! I re-taught myself how to use my new hand and arm. I taught myself to fish again in a new way. My wife and I were getting use to my new normal quality of life. It was not great but it was a huge improvement from where I had been. The meds were managing it enough I went back to work, I was fishing again, and I felt a sense of self-worth again. I could bathe and dress myself again, all the things that I had taken for granted. Then, the CDC and the DEA came in with their new guidelines and scared my doctor and he cut me off immediately without a word or reason.

He refused to transfer me to another doctor or even see me. I have not seen a doctor in over two years or had any pain relief in that long, and I am back at square one, as some days I still cannot use my hand or arm or I will go into a huge flare-up.

CRPS is a beast in and of itself, yet I also have severe joint pain, arthritis, and phantom limb pain.

I have found that Medical cannabis has been an important part of my treatment. I have found it helps the mental side of things, so I can handle the physical side of my CRPS.

73

I'm asked a lot how do I keep going every day, and I respond I have no choice. I have to keep going or I will die. Please do not ever give up, even though it is so easy too. I lost all of my most important relationships because of this monster, along with so many other things. You have to keep pushing! My wife is still here and I do not know why? I guess she truly loves me.

My advice to anyone going through the CRPS circus is to be your own advocate. Fight for your human rights! Research thoroughly any treatment plan, and finally never give up! Stay strong warriors!

Making Lemonade
Robin Brueckmann

I developed complex regional pain syndrome (CRPS) after a simple slip and fall on ice in early February 1994. I tore my Tarsometatarsal (TMT) joint on my right foot, and it did not heal well. I had instability in the joint which exacerbated my pain. My foot was black for months, and eventually, it was black during the day but fairly normal colored when elevated. I had around 30 procedures the first year to try to reset the nerves, different kinds of blocks in my back, Bier block, epidural space, and around the spine, including a parasympathetic catheter for three months.

Meanwhile, I was working at my regular job, teaching horseback riding, and also working on upgrading my judge's license. This entailed apprenticing at 26 different horse shows, all over the country, as well as judging my normal roster of horse shows. I could not ride my horse, though, which was devastating to me.

I saw a number of different doctors. I went to two different pain clinics in Pennsylvania, Thomas Jefferson Hospital in Philadelphia, and Brandywine Hospital in Chester county. I saw a neurologist, three different orthopedists in Pennsylvania and one in North Carolina, as well as my original doctor, a podiatrist. I was in a splint or cast or an AFO from 1994 until my amputation in 2011 and was unable to bear weight on my forefoot for the duration until my amputation.

My judge's license was approved, and I continued to be an active judge, traveling all over the country judging dressage shows and horse trials. I returned to riding in 1995, although I could not tolerate pressure from stirrups. I was severely debilitated, and very grateful for my horse with whom I already had a solid relationship. He tolerated my asymmetry and allowed me to regain strength and balance as I could.

We moved to NC in 1996, and I started seeing a different pain clinic physician and different orthopedist. This orthopedist was willing to do surgery to correct the extreme contractures I had developed. He did an Achilles release, plantar fascia release, calcaneal osteotomy, and midfoot fusion, and put me into a PTB brace once I healed from the surgery. This surgery relieved the mechanical pain that I had, although the CRPS was still active.

Because I was not allowed to compete, I started doing exhibitions instead. My wonderful horse allowed me to ride him without a bridle, and I did exhibitions of international-level freestyles without a bridle. I wrote a book about our relationship, titled When Two Are One. Even though I could not compete, I could do things with my horse that no one else could do.

In 1998, I had an indwelling epidural catheter installed, running Clonidine 24/7. This did give me some relief. It was awkward riding with a pump and bag of juice, but I managed it.

Because I rode without stirrups, I was not permitted to compete at national-level shows. I did get Classified as a Para rider. I was classified as an amputee, even though I was not yet, on the basis of the trophic changes and paralysis resulting from CRPS. I started competing internationally and won two Gold Medals and a Bronze at the Dressage World Championships in Denmark in 1999. I competed in the Sydney Paralympics in 2000, World Championships in Belgium in 2003, shortlisted for Athens Paralympics in 2004, rode in World Championships in England in 2007, and competed at the Beijing Paralympics in 2008. I competed in the World Equestrian Games in Kentucky in 2010 and was short-listed for the London

Paralympics in 2012. Now I am a Selector, currently watching riders aiming for the 2021 Tokyo Paralympics. I have filled that role since 2014.

I did receive permission to compete without stirrups and returned to national-level competition in 1999. Since then, I have earned numerous Horse of the Year awards, on multiple horses, at all levels.

I finally got my orthopedist to agree that I might find better mobility with an amputation. He referred me to a colleague who mostly treats diabetics, and is very experienced with amputations. He performed a trans-tibial amputation in November 2011. I was home in three days and started outpatient physical therapy at seven-weeks post-surgery after I was fitted for a prosthesis. My recovery was good, although my PT wanted me to be very cautious; she did not want me to force progress and potentially go back into CRPS pain. Twelve weeks after surgery, I drove my horse 15-hours to Wellington, FL to compete in a Qualifier for London, and there I did get my Certificate of Capability to allow me to continue the qualifying process.

Since my amputation, I have become fully functional again. I use crutches at night only. When I have breeches or long pants on, no one can tell that I have an amputation. I have an app on my phone that registers gait irregularity, and I am consistently under 2% irregular, which is consistent with a prosthetic ankle. I am free of all CRPS pain. I ride my horse every day, teach lessons, and judge horse shows without any physical limitations. Life is good.

A LITTLE ABOUT MY CRPS
Elizabeth Kaftan

It all started for me when I was a runner with bunions. So, like many, I had bunion surgery, and subtalar implants placed in my ankles, in 2016 for my right foot, and 2017 for the left foot.

Unfortunately, something just was not right with my right foot, which started becoming more painful every day and affecting my sleep. My Podiatrist starting treating me for a neuroma, which, unfortunately, was not the root cause of my pain.

I decided to get a second opinion as I continued getting worse. Doctor H.C., who diagnosed me with complex regional pain syndrome (CRPS), sent me to pain management and continued to make sure that my pain management doctors were taking good care of me. They did an amazing job trying so hard to help my pain, with Gabapentin, Flexeril, and a spinal cord stimulator (SCS) in November 2019.

Unfortunately, that did not work, and I was having issues with my heart and had to now see a cardiologist, who had to treat me with Kapspargo Sprinkle for my blood pressure. I had stress tests and found out that it seemed my high blood pressure and tachycardia were due to my foot pain. The Cardiology said that it had to be controlled somehow.

Every day I struggled with the fight to survive the lack of sleep, the pain, and the fact that I could not even wear shoes due to pain or even cut my toenails.

I was very blessed with having huge support from my co-workers and witnessing me slowly having more and more trouble walking on that foot.

78

I had started getting sores, with a couple of infections I just had treated by an urgent care doctor.

I kept remembering the conversation I had with Doctor H.C., about possibly amputation if my pain could not be controlled. I believe that conversation is what kept me alive, because that was a potential solution before, I did something extreme like take my life.

I will say I had an amazing caring team with Doctor H.C., who performed a right below-knee (BK) amputation on September 3, 2020.

When I woke up Doctor H.C., was there to make sure I was okay, and when he showed me it was gone, I was so happy. My pain was so minimal and completely gone now.

I'm currently awaiting my definitive socket, but was able to do three to four-plus miles on my test socket, which in four-years was huge!!!

I no longer need any medications and since the day of my amputation, my blood pressure and heart rate are completely normal again, and I am finally sleeping again.

While amputation is not the right choice for everyone, it was the right choice for me, and this is giving me the chance to be active again with running and hiking with my dogs, so I'm extremely happy at my second chance in life to do that.

THE DRUNK DRIVER LOST HER LIFE, CHANGED MY LIFE FOREVER AND SHE WAS MY MOTHER: MY LIFE WITH COMPLEX REGIONAL PAIN SYNDROME (CRPS)

Tabatha Carter

On August 9, 1988, it was a hot summer day, and I was supposed to be celebrating my 6th birthday. We were at a friend's farm, that was just south of town to celebrate and to have a sleepover with my friends, but sometime later during the evening, there was an argument between some adults outside that had been drinking. My mother came in and said it was time to go, and you can imagine my attitude towards her as I wanted a sleepover with my friends; I mean, it was my birthday party after all. Most children do not win an argument like this, so ultimately, I ended up in the back of our car with our dog, and we started driving down the driveway. My mother and her friend were arguing in the front seat, the last thing I remember was asking her to please slow down. I am not sure how much time went by, but when I awoke it seemed to be so bright with everything inside the car illuminating even though it was the middle of the night, there was broken glass everywhere and I called out to my mother who was slouched over the steering wheel just starring in my direction and her friend was halfway on the hood and half still inside the vehicle. So much fear consumed me. What just happened? Why does my mother look like that? Why is there blood everywhere? Where did all this glass come from? I opened my door to get out and stepped out, and I fell to the ground and the pain just took over my body, and started crying for help. Why are we at the bottom of the ditch? Why am I in so much pain? I had no idea my leg was fractured in several places and when I tried to step out of the vehicle, one of the sharp broken bones pierced through my skin. I crawled up the side of the ditch and I saw a pickup truck coming down the driveway, luckily my dog had run back to the farm, which alerted them something had gone horribly wrong so they called 911 and came down to help while waiting for the ambulance to arrive. It all seemed to happen so fast after that, the ambulance showed up and took me and my mother's friend in the same ambulance, but why wasn't I with my mother? Why did they leave her behind? I remember asking for my mother over and over and over and no one would tell me a thing. It wasn't until later my father told me that my mother died on impact. I've had to relive this night over and over in my dreams, the pain and fear would feel so real and no one ever really asked why I would wake up screaming, I can only assume they already knew why. The nightmares lessened over time but never went away.

I was not diagnosed with complex regional pain syndrome (CRPS) until later on in life. I had multiple surgeries to repair my left leg, I was hospitalized for a length of time for them to perform all the surgeries, I even had to miss my mother's funeral. I spent a few months in a wheelchair and eventually started working with physical therapy and later graduated to crutches and eventually I was walking and running on my own. I did well for several years after, I even played in several sports throughout high school before my life was flipped upside down again. One summer morning in 2008, I awoke to my left leg so swollen and painful I could not even bear any weight on that leg. This is where my journey with CRPS started it was believed that over time the nerve endings were, I had to have skin grafts, became aggravated over time, I had always been very sensitive to anything touching my skin grafts to the point where no one, including myself, was able to touch that area and that area was right where my shoe would constantly rub. I just did not and still do not understand to this day, how I could go from being completely "normal" for 20 years with no pain, except for the sensitivity on the grafts, and no swelling, to the most horrific pain one can endure.

TRYING TO FIND A DIAGNOSIS

Trying to find a reason for the swelling and pain with no known injury was so exhausting, it felt like I was bouncing from doctor to doctor and test after test. You start to feel like no one believes you, but, how couldn't they? My leg was extremely swollen and discolored. I had so many different scans done, X-rays, CT, MRI, Ultrasounds and Nuclear Bone Scans all ordered by several different doctors, rheumatologists, neurologists, pain specialists, and my primary doctor. After what felt like years but was only a year, I was diagnosed with reflex sympathetic dystrophy (RSD), which is now known as complex regional pain syndrome (CRPS) and I was told there was no cure but treatment can help. During this time, I had been taking pain medications that did not take the pain away but helped decrease the intensity of the pain. I started on gabapentin on top of the pain medications as it was shown to help neuropathic pain. It seemed to take some of the edge off but the side effects were horrible. I was trying to finish college and raise three children but I was tired and in pain constantly. My pain specialist had recommended trying some nerve blocks which seem to only aggravate my symptoms and with my blood pressure so low I have issues with fainting after so I elected to stop the blocks. My pain specialist had recommended doing physical therapy which I have done on and off throughout the years as I could afford it. I was able to push through my pain and finish college but had to be on oral pain meds and anticonvulsants and wearing a compression sock on that leg all day every day to control swelling.

In 2016, the pain started increasing out of the blue no injury or anything that would explain the aggravated symptoms. I tried more nerve blocks, different medications, even trial medications that were still being trial phases. My pain specialist recommended implanting a spinal cord stimulator, with my pain running 6-8/10 every day and the blocks and medications failing I elected to try the spinal cord stimulator (SCS). I did the trial and had a decrease in pain so the permanent SCS was implanted which decreased my pain levels down to 3-5/10 pain level, I was still on oral pain meds and gabapentin with the SCS but the combo seemed to help. Then in 2018, once again there was a huge spike in pain and other health issues arose. They found that my peripheral nerve in my left leg wasn't responding the same anymore and was causing my foot drop so they ordered an AFO in hopes to prevent me from tripping so much. It was recommended to try an intrathecal pain pump, the trial was an injection of morphine in the spine which left me unable to urinate on my own, I had to place a urinary catheter in myself over the next 12-24 hours to empty my bladder. Since there was a reduction of pain the intrathecal pump was implanted and I would just start on a lower dose of morphine, my pain doctor thought that the reason I was unable to urinate was because it was a larger dose all at once and the intrathecal pump would give smaller amounts throughout the day. Well, he could not have been more wrong, I spent the next few weeks struggling to urinate and I was dizzy and nauseous.

The morphine was taken out and replaced with hydromorphone. I started getting dizzy and nauseous all the time, they did not think it was from the medications and said it was likely dehydration. As the time went on, I noticed that I was more constipated than normal and struggled to pass a bowel movement to the point I ended up having a uterus prolapse which resulted in me having a hysterectomy. I went home the same day after my hysterectomy but started having intense pain later that night so bad I went into the ER and they found a softball size blood clot in my abdomen, I was bleeding internally. I spent the next week in the hospital but made a full recovery. The months passed on and I kept getting sicker and sicker, I was passing out having heart palpitations and hypoglycemia and was eventually hospitalized. After running several tests, they found that I had adrenal insufficiency and my liver isn't storing glycogen anymore. I met with a diabetic nutritionist on how to regulate my blood sugar by eating foods that store sugar longer, wear a continuous glucose monitor that alerts me when I am going too low. I was started on steroids for my adrenal insufficiency. It is believed all of this is related to the intrathecal pump giving me continuous hydromorphone all day and or from long-term opioid use prior. During all this time my pain was out of control, so I was sick all day every day and, in more pain, than anyone could ever feel. After all, this was figured out, I went back to my pain specialist who recommended trying a peripheral nerve stimulator, they injected lidocaine along my peripheral nerve and what do you know for roughly about an hour or two I had really good pain relief, my leg felt warm again so the peripheral nerve stimulator was implanted.

So, imagine this: I wake up in the morning, put my compression sock on, then my AFO for my foot drop, then this battery and antenna is wrapped around that. I would turn the SCS on, the intrathecal pump already going, turn the peripheral stim on, eat and take my steroid and what do you know no reduction of pain, my pain was still getting worse. Then over the last summer, I started having significant pain in my right foot, I could barely walk, I was in so much pain. I got a referral to podiatry and they found I had a torn spring ligament and my bone was deformed causing an adult flat foot which is believed to be from my gait and overuse of that leg since it was my good leg and I was avoiding bearing weight on my left. This is when I said I am done, I just cannot do this anymore, I want to amputate. I was able to get a referral to a vascular surgeon where he did a few tests to rule out some things that had not yet been looked at and what do you know there was peripheral artery disease and the lesion on my bone had bone loss and severe muscle atrophy. He said we would be willing to amputate in light of these and in the hope to alleviate my pain.

AMPUTATION

My amputation was December 3, 2020, and when I woke up from surgery, I think I was a little dysphoric or in shock not sure which but within a few hours my pain had decreased and within 24 hours I was pain-free. I have had no phantom pain or sensations and my physical therapist says I am exceeding his expectations. I am working on improving my strength and balance and looking forward to hopefully one day soon be in a prosthetic. While I know everything is new and things can change, I have a very positive attitude and a renewed outlook on life. I feel like I was taken from the brink of death and revived back to life. Living with CRPS is in my opinion one of the worst conditions to live with, there is a reason it's called "The suicide disease" as many of us living with it constantly think about it as we see it as our only way out. I hope to raise more awareness of this very poorly understood disease in hopes to find a treatment that actually works and eventually a cure for CRPS.

THE KILLER DISEASE THAT CHANGED MY LIFE

Shawn O'Brien

In January 2018, I had a work-related injury from a skid falling off a forklift that hit me on the soft part of my left shoulder, and it cracked a bone. The damage was not enough to have surgery, so we thought it would heal on its own.

A month later my left arm and hand started to swell up, and it kept on getting bigger and bigger. The doctor I was seeing at the time said it looked like I had complex regional pain syndrome (CRPS), but he was not too sure about the diagnosis?

Then this doctor had referred me to see a pain specialist. I went to see Doctor B., and she recommended that I try the Ketamine I.V. infusion. She had recommended that I do four of these infusions.

The first Ketamine infusion made me feel so drugged up, I slept for six hours. It was the best sleep I had since I was diagnosed with CRPS. For the next three months, I had the Ketamine infusion again, which provided me with no pain relief.

After seeing Doctor B., I went to see another pain specialist Doctor G., had mentioned to me that he wanted to try a drug that they only had enough for three patients, and he was hoping that this would work for me, but unfortunately, it did not work. I had a very bad reaction to this drug.

So, now they did not know what to do with me. The doctor had sent me to Physiotherapy and after four months of physio, my arm and hand were getting bigger. My physiotherapist found a therapist who specializes in CRPS. He worked on me for over one year and nothing worked for me. He suggested that the best thing for me was amputation, so we found a surgeon in Toronto, Canada who said he would do the amputation.

When I went to see this surgeon, he wanted to do more tests before he did the amputation. So, he had sent me for a bone scan, and another MRI, which I could not do because of the size of my arm. It would not fit into the MRI machine. The technician tried for about one hour, but could not do it without hurting me. Then I was sent for a CT scan and x-rays.

After having these tests, I went back to see the doctor, and he said to me, I am going to send you to see another pain specialist in Toronto, and then he would make his decision.

So back to Toronto, I went for the third time. The Doctor came in and said to me that I have three options we can try.

- The first option was doing the Ketamine infusion.
- The second option was doing the spinal cord simulator (SCS).
- The third option took him awhile, but I told him amputation.

 I felt that amputation was the best option for me because the Ketamine infusion did not work and as far as the SCS was concerned it was not happening. So, we decided to amputate.

The doctor had sent his report to the surgeon. So, I went back to see the surgeon, and he decided not to do the surgery and told me he wanted to do more tests. I got mad and told him that I was tired of being a guinea pig and doing more tests was not going to happen. He had the nerve to tell me that I was faking this and to see him in two years and then maybe he will amputate.

Thank God, I was seeing a psychologist because on my way out of his office I had to make an appointment to see him as I was going to snap. I see Doctor K., once a week or as many times as I need to.

Now, it is December of 2019, and again, I had to find a surgeon who would do the amputation. I found one in London. Doctor R., who is a plastic surgeon and the way my arm was I was doing this for my health. Doctor R., had me sign all kinds of papers to have the amputation done. Now I was just waiting for Doctor R., to call me with the surgery date. I received the call and my surgery was scheduled for March 13, 2020. At this time, I had CRPS for two-years.

Doctor R., told me that I would be the first person in Canada to have a Trans-radial amputation from CRPS. On the day of the surgery, they did a sympathetic nerve block to try and stop the CRPS from spreading after the surgery.

As for me, my life was about to change after I woke up from the surgery. The surgery lasted about ninety minutes, but I was in recovery for three hours. When I got to my room I was scared to look so, my wife showed me on my right arm how much was amputated. So, now we are into March 14th the next day, the surgeon who worked with Doctor R., came in and took off the bandages to see it and I asked him to take a picture of it and when I was ready, I would look at it.

The surgeon waited until my wife and kids were in the room to tell us that if the arm was not amputated when they did it, the surgeon said I might have lasted a month before I died because the arm was so far gone. They had never seen anything like this before. My arm had to be doubled bagged to be disposed of.

I spent three days in the hospital and seven days in a hotel before I was allowed to go home, and at this time COVID-19 started. Now it is March 21, and I am now home. My new life begins with one arm and no more CRPS.

In July 2020, I started having a difficult time with my amputation, that I tried to commit suicide, but I thought about my wife, my family, and close friends on how they would go on without me and I stopped.

In November, I did a news story on CRPS to help people and more Doctors to understand that CRPS is no joke, and one day I would like to be an advocate to help other CRPS patients.

Now it is nine months later and my CRPS is back, not only do I have to deal with the amputation I have to deal with CRPS all over again. I used to be an outdoor person now I do not leave my home. I now suffer from panic attacks and my house is my safe zone.

I thank my wife for being with me through all of this. She deserves a medal for this. On really bad days I go to that dark spot in my brain. I have a saying on the fridge that my wife gave me. It says **"I cannot lose you, because if I ever did, I'd have lost my best friend, my soul mate, my smile, my laugh, my everything."** This stops me.

I am still seeing my psychiatrist, and when I cannot talk to him, I call my brother from another mother, Philip he also helps me quite a bit at times. Philip might as well be my psychiatrist. Lol!

Now that my CRPS is back I am helping a friend I met in London who also has CRPS and Philip's 11-year-old who has it in his feet.

So, if I was not around, they would not have anyone to lean, on and they would have to fight this battle on their own.

So, no matter how much pain I am in I go one day at a time to fight this horrible disease they call the suicide disease and learn how to do stuff with my one arm. I now joke that my wife is my left arm and I love her for it.

Thank you for letting me tell my story.

MY FUN TIME AT THE BEACH CAUSED MY CRPS

JoAnne Cohen

My name is JoAnne and my complex regional pain syndrome (CRPS) was caused by a left ankle reconstruction surgery that I had on October 25, 1987. This all started when I had injured my left ankle the in the summer of 1986, while I was in Ocean City, New Jersey.

I had been given a pair of orthotics which weakened my ankles. I took a shortcut to the ocean, which I never thought twice about. I was jumping from the bulkhead onto the wet sand and right into the ocean. When I jumped down, I did not feel any pain. When I came out of the ocean, my left ankle was stinging, and swollen and I could not remember what I could have possibly done to have injured my ankle. I kept up with my friends and kept walking on it for about a month. I was experiencing a lot of pain and eventually, my ankle kept twisting on me. I was headed back to Ocean City for a week's vacation, and I had no intentions of seeing an Orthopedic Surgeon until after my good time was over. I did not want to stop having a good time, in other words. I had no choice but the end of August before Labor Day weekend I forced by the pain I had incurred to be seen.

I was sent for an x-ray before being seen and when I was seen I was told I had a seriously sprained ankle and needed to be fitted with an air cast. I wore that for a while and then needed more support, so they applied a walking cast for six to eight weeks. I went to physical therapy (PT) to strengthen the ankle, but it was not helping. At that time, it was determined that I need further imaging, and I was so scared because the orthopedic surgeon performing the test was not one to have bedside manners. Anytime I asked a question out of fear, he seemed annoyed. I had a test that entailed shooting air through a syringe that was put right into the ankle bone joint. That was supposed to give them a better idea what kind of ligament damage I had. An x-ray could not see this, but this painful test could.

I survived it but after speaking to my father about he wished I went to another hospital for better care. It was determined that my ankle ligaments were pulled and stretched so much from not being properly attended to from the first initial point of injury that probably would have saved a lot of stressful situations. The situation goes into another topic of discussion and that is surgical repair, which was something I was not a happy camper about. I saw another orthopedic surgeon over in Philadelphia, and he came on strong and again had a terrible bedside manner. I again saw another orthopedic surgeon in Maryland, and he reconfirmed what the first orthopedic surgeon said was ligament reconstruction, and at that point, I was so scared that I sought another opinion. This orthopedic surgeon went into detail about what it involved, and I had it done. I did well with the surgery. The hard part was the rehabilitation, which was twice a week for six months.

When I developed CRPS, I did not know what this was. My family thought it had a connection with Muscular Dystrophy until we found out through my cousin who was in the medical field knew of someone who dealt with it as well. I had intense PT which included ice and heat treatments, and whirlpool therapy, and tens unit stimulation.

I had serious swelling because I had to wear a cast shoe for close to six months until the swelling went down, and I could wear my regular shoe and sneaker. It felt like an eternity for me and hell. As time went on, the PT was cut back to once a week for a month and then I was finally cut loose. For once in my life, I felt a lot better and could go back out and play tennis, drive without hesitation and go to work. I never wanted to experience that again. I was very fortunate to have the CRPS go away for good.

I had an injury to my right ankle not too long after recovering from ankle reconstructive surgery and Physical Therapy. I had twisted my right ankle unfortunately in my driveway we just had a major ice storm and of course, my ankles were weakened from the orthotics that were prescribed which ruined my ankles in the long run.

I had many surgeries and a lot of letdowns and recurring staph infections, Hickman catheters, which I could not stand. My brother put the bug in my ear about considering amputation of my right ankle. He said JoAnne, I do not think you want to keep getting cut and not being able to live a normal life. The light bulb went on in my head and I thought seriously about it. I said to myself; I need to go think this over and do more research on it.

Even though I went through a lot with my left ankle, I was thinking about what will my mom and dad say to this. My brother said do not worry, I will talk to Dad about this and explain why you went this route. My brother was in the service and was a medic in the Army. He was in Desert Storm and saw a lot of limbs loss amongst servicemen and women. He also had to pick up severed limbs off the front lines after fighting the war. My father was very anxious that the chronic osteomyelitis I had would spread up my leg to my knee.

The same orthopedic surgeon that came highly recommended to me was the one that did the amputation. He was the most honest and reassuring orthopedic surgeon I had ever had. Many people I consulted with knew of him and his knowledge of doing amputations and dealing with chronic osteomyelitis. I had my father come to one pre-op visits to hear the orthopedic surgeon's questions and answers to my upcoming amputation.

My father admitted he did not want his daughter to become an invalid, and the orthopedic surgeon said to him that he felt my outcome will be a success, even though I had twenty unsuccessful surgeries. My father was reassured that the osteomyelitis would not spread because the amputation would prevent this from happening.

I was able to keep my knee which is a given because I can have stability, so I can have some good balance with my prosthetic limb. My mom had a lot of knowledge of osteomyelitis because she worked at a nursing college and had all sources of information at her fingertips. She knew I would be better off, and I have proved it to my family, friends, coworkers, and strangers.

I had the amputation on January 8, 2002, which I was ready for and could not wait for the date to come. I even wrote a message in a sharpie marker on my right leg for my orthopedic surgeon and his team. It said please take this leg and not the left. I know the orthopedic surgeon knew to take the right one it had a wide-open wound in the ankle bone. The left one did not. I have read mark the correct body part to be removed in case of taking the wrong body part. When I showed my mom and dad, they said you are being overly cautious. I was wheeled into the operating room and off to sleep, I went after going over the usual questions of making sure I am who I am on the wrist bracelet and what I was having done.

I think my amputation was close to four hours and when I woke up, I was surrounded by wonderful nurses. The most important person I wanted to see was my dad to tell him I did well with the amputation. My mom was anxious to see me as well because she knew I made the best decision to get rid of this mess.

I know my orthopedic surgeon sat with me for a long while to make sure I felt comfortable. I was able to say to him, it is late please go home, I feel comfortable being here. I think he knew I had fear inside me because of the discussions we had with him and how I was advised to just imagine myself one step at a time being without my limb, and then seeing the amputated stump in the orthopedic clinic before I left the hospital three days later.

A hard cast was applied. I told the orthopedic surgeon how scared I was about the unavailing of this site. He offered to prescribe something to calm me down before I am wheeled to the orthopedic clinic. I said yes, I think that would help me. I felt a calming sensation come over me which did help me a lot. I was on my way to becoming a mobile person again after the amputation. I still had much work to do. I had a fast PT class in the hospital on the day of discharge, how to go up and down steps with crutches. What to do if you fall and how to get up which I thought would be easy but was not.

I was pretty fortunate my orthopedic surgeon decided to let me go home to my bed and home. Instead of going by way of medical transport to a rehabilitation center. He felt very different because of my situation. My physical therapy sessions were two times a week for four weeks, and then I had a follow-up. I was doing very well at that point, and I was in touch with a prosthetist. I did a lot of interviewing of prosthetic companies before the amputation happened. I had a lot of time on my hands. I also joined an amputee support group early on and also attended meetings up until the amputation. I needed to speak to amputees who went through this first hand and listen to their stories. It made me feel more comfortable about what I was facing. I met many people young and old. I kept attending the amputee meetings for many years and finally, my life changed, and I did not need their help.

I also joined an adaptive sports group in Philadelphia. I did adaptive bike riding, rowing. I also have tried kayaking in recent years, but my sport is tennis which I have been playing since the age of 6-years-old. I did not want to lose that skill I have had all these years. I eventually joined an organization that had a tennis clinic and turned into playing round robins. I think having all these experiences throughout my life was a wake-up call when it came to undergoing twenty unsuccessful surgeries and then deciding amputation is what I needed to do to get on with my life.

I also reached out to a psychiatrist for mental help dealing with the situation I was in. I still see him every month, and it does help. As an amputee, you face many situations and need guidance on how to get through it. Many people have no idea what a catastrophic injury is until they experience it themselves. I think I have overcome a lot, but the fear is still out there in some way for me being an amputee.

I have a saying as well that helped me. You can do anything you want as long as you put your mind to it and do not let anyone tell you cannot do it because you can. It is a proven fact with myself and when I tell people this saying, they look at me. I feel it does help when you think about it. Always remember you are a fighter and not a quitter as I say. I always tell people this too.

Good luck and hang in there.

STEVEN'S CRPS AND AMPUTATION STORY
Steven Tighe

My complex regional pain syndrome (CRPS) journey started on June 10, 2018, when I broke my right leg while skateboarding. I had broken the fibula which is the hardest bone to break. My wife had taken me to the hospital, and they confirmed the break. A couple of days later, I had an appointment to see Doctor T.L. an orthopedic surgeon.

Doctor T.L. informed me I needed surgery to fix my leg, so I had scheduled the surgery. Doctor T.L. put a plate and seven screws in my leg. I could not wear the walking boot, because the weight of the walking boot was weighing my leg off to the side where I had the hardware. It was making my leg hurt more.

A week after my surgery, I had to call the doctor's office to get a refill on my pain medication, which should have been a warning that I was in a lot of pain. The sad thing is the doctor would not believe me, and he thought I was playing the system. My foot was already changing color, and it became more swollen.

Seven weeks after my surgery, the doctor finally referred me to see Doctor G, a pain specialist. When I went to see Doctor G, she did her tests and confirmed I had CRPS type II. Both Doctor T.L. and Doctor G, suggested I do physical therapy (PT) and try some medications to help control the pain. Also, I did not have any bracing to protect my leg.

Around September or October, I fell off my porch with my crutches and landed on my CRPS foot and I heard a loud pop. My wife rushed me back to the hospital to make sure there were no broken bones, or I did not ruin the surgery.

A few months went by, and Doctor T.L., informed me that there was nothing more he could do for me, and he threw his hands up. Also, Doctor G was giving me the runaround too. Our insurance had stopped the PT because it was not helping me. My wife was not working because she had to take care of me.

Doctor G wanted me to get a cell phone we could not afford at all. She wanted me to use an App that would help control my CRPS. My wife and I started looking for other doctors for a second opinion. One doctor I saw said I was the perfect candidate for amputation, and the other doctors said no to having an amputation.

In December 2018, I finally found Doctor W, a podiatrist. He had performed two surgeries to fix the nerves. I saw him until October 2019.

In November 2019, my wife and I moved to Maine because I could not find any doctor to treat me. My foot was dropping significantly, and my foot would turn purple and would be cold to the touch.

In 2020, I finally found a great team of doctors could help me. In May 2020, I had a right below-knee amputation (BKA). I also found a great prosthetist J.V. from Hanger Prosthetics, who has been working with me to get me walking again. So far, he has made me four prosthetics. I now have a mechanical foot, and I am no longer in pain.

I am thankful to the State of Maine and all of my doctors!

POEM

PHANTOM PAIN

(A.K.A. "THE PHANTOM")

Eric M. Phillips

PHANTOM PAIN YOU WAKE ME FROM A DEEP SLEEP WITH YOUR UNRELENTING STABBING PAIN.

PHANTOM PAIN YOU KEEP ME UP FOR HOURS ON END

PHANTOM PAIN YOU ARE SO STRONG THAT PAIN MEDS DON'T PHASE YOU AT ALL

PHANTOM PAIN YOU COME TO REMIND ME OF MY OLD PAINFUL LIMB THAT HAS BEEN GONE FOR SO LONG

PHANTOM PAIN YOUR UNRELENTING PAIN GOES ON AND ON

PHANTOM PAIN YOU ROBB ME OF MY PRECIOUS TIME AND SLEEP

PHANTOM PAIN YOUR RELENTLESS PAIN SEEMS TO NEVER END AND I KNOW THAT IT'S NOT IN MY HEAD

PHANTOM PAIN I FIGHT WITH YOU FOR HOURS ON END, BUT I KNOW THAT I WILL WIN IN THE END

CRPS INFORMATION RESOURCE PAGE

CRPS education and awareness are very important to patients and their family members.

Through education, awareness, and research may be someday we can find a cure for CRPS?

For more helpful information on CRPS, please visit The International RSD Foundation at:

www.rsdinfo.com

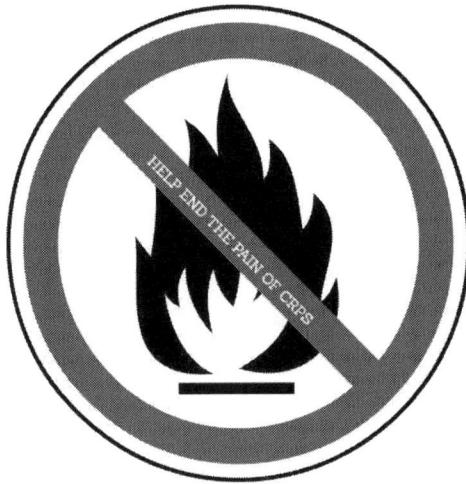